MIND
&
BOWL

LAURENCE KING

First published in Great Britain in 2022
by Laurence King Publishing an imprint
of The Orion Publishing Group Ltd
Carmelite House, 50 Victoria Embankment
London EC4Y 0DZ

An Hachette UK Company

10 9 8 7 6 5 4 3 2 1

© Text 2022 Joey Hulin
Illustrations by Awu Iwashima

A CIP catalogue record for this book is
available from the British Library.

ISBN: 978-1-39960-006-4

Printed in China by C&C Offset Printing Co., Ltd.
Laurence King Publishing is committed to ethical
and sustainable production. We are proud participants of The Book Chain Project
bookchainproject.com

www.laurenceking.com
www.orionbooks.co.uk

A GUIDE TO MINDFUL EATING & COOKING

MIND & BOWL

JOEY HULIN

Illustrations by Awu Iwashima

Contents

Introduction

first wrote this book as a pocket guide for guests who attend the well-being retreats I host in Cornwall, South West England. At the end of each retreat, guests would ask for the recipes of meals they had enjoyed—often meat-eaters surprised at how much they appreciated a mostly plant-based menu. I am not a professionally trained chef or a nutritionist, but I do love to cook, and I am fascinated by the topics we will investigate together in this book. Through my work exploring meditation, spirituality, and creativity, I am on a mission to understand how the mind manifests our experiences, physical health, and general well-being.

Food, eating, and our own personal relationship to our body are topics that can be highly sensitive and deeply personal and this book seeks to honor the uniqueness and individuality of us all. There is no "one way," no "right way," or quick fix. What is right for me may not be right for you, but what a mindful eating practice encourages us to do is to lovingly become aware of who, what, and where we are, without judgment.

This is not a book about dieting or weight loss. It isn't about turning vegan, never eating chocolate again, or offering dietary advice. Nor is it about producing flawless, Michelin-style meals that require exotic, never-before-heard-of, "how do you spell that again?" ingredients. It is a book about self-awareness, self-care and playing with the idea that the food we eat is part of an intimate relationship between us and the earth. This book is simply offering you an opportunity to mindfully explore your own habits and relationship with food and offer you inspiration for creating your own bowls of colorful, plant-based goodness.

I hope reading this book will feel comforting, practical, and inspiring, while creating an opportunity for you to refresh your relationship with food. I believe paying attention to how and what we eat offers us subtle clues about our relationship to self and to the earth. Mindful eating is an opportunity to witness and lovingly explore our habits and choices, as a way of deepening a wider sense of self-awareness, self-love, and connection. The plant-based recipes included are for simple, uncomplicated, home-cooked meals which I make myself on retreats. Have some fun creating these colorful bowls of goodness and sharing that joy with others. You are encouraged to play with, experiment with, and adapt the recipes to make them your own. Be sure to share your creations and reflections with me on Instagram by tagging @joeyhulin_writer #mindandbowl.

The retreats and meditation I offer carry a very simple intention: to create a nourishing, down-to-earth, and welcoming space for people to pause and reconnect. Often, spending time on retreat enables people to experience subtle shifts in how they both feel inside themselves and view the world. I hope you see this book as an opportunity to do just that, wherever you are.

Because—look!—this book is in your hands and, as with all things, there will be a reason why we are here together, at this time. Whether you are looking for a friendly hand to hold as you explore something new or a mindset shift when it comes to your relationship with food, I am so glad you are here.

Consider this little book a permission slip: to pause, reflect, and maybe start letting yourself believe that you are exactly who, what, and where you're meant to be. You have the power of choice, to move forward in a direction that feels truly right and loving for you and the planet. I hope this book will inspire you to find joy, balance, and creativity in your relationship with food and within yourself.

So, here's to eating food, glorious food, and to savoring every single bite.

CHAPTER ONE

MINDFULNESS AND MINDFUL EATING

Mindfulness is more than just a buzzword. It is true to say, though, that the widely discussed yet rarely embodied practice of being present in the moment often comes cloaked in confusion. I remember the first mindfulness session I ever attended, led by a trained psychologist turned mindfulness teacher. A small group of us were instructed to sit in a circle, close our eyes and take a few deep breaths. We were each handed a raisin and told to look at it, smell it, and taste the tiniest little nibble before being given permission to eat it. I remember sitting there, darting my eyes from side to side, scanning the circle of concentrated faces to see if anyone else thought the exercise was completely embarrassing and pointless. I left the session thinking: "What a load of nonsense!" and went on about my day, consumed by thoughts, judgments, and unconscious habits.

In my experience, embracing mindfulness requires a series of pennies to drop, one after another. The subtle shift in perception that a committed mindfulness practice brings about moves us from thinking to feeling—doing to being—and from living in our heads to living in our hearts. The practice of mindfulness requires us to wake up and realize we are not our thoughts or feelings; they are simply something we experience.

But try to tell someone who completely identifies with their thoughts and feelings that those thoughts are not reality: It is frustrating, confusing, and utterly irritating for them. I know because I was one of those people. "How can you say I'm not my thoughts or feelings? I don't even understand what that means," I would think to myself, followed by "They don't know what it's like to be me."

Back then I would sleepwalk my way through each day in a foggy, automated headspace. I'd wake up in the morning tired after a poor, broken night's sleep, and reach for my phone for a

> # "To practice mindfulness is to be deliberately present in our experiences"

quick scroll in search of my self-worth. I would stagger my way to the shower, barely conscious, where I'd begin to worry about the day ahead and start running a narrative in my mind of how busy and stressed I was. My mind would replay memories of the past, mentally transporting me to a different time and place, inciting feelings of anxiety or longing in that moment, there in the shower. I'd slurp coffee and eat breakfast on the go, staying in that foggy headspace on my drive to work, often arriving at my destination with no real recollection of the journey there. I'd spend the day with my eyes fixed on a computer screen. I'd eat lunch at my desk and hardly take a single physical or mental break. I'd sometimes go to the gym after work, remaining in my head as I turned up the speed on the treadmill to go faster and faster. Without any thought or consideration, I would make something quick for dinner and consume it on the sofa with my attention on the television. A couple of glasses of wine later, I'd head up to bed, only to sleep badly—and around the cycle would go again.

To practice mindfulness is to be deliberately present in our experiences, as we are experiencing them—in the moment. When you take your morning shower, are your body and mind really in the shower? Is your mind in the fantasy world of thought and your body in a state of anxiety or stress? To be present would be to feel the sensation of the water on your skin, to savor the fragrance of the soap, to notice what is right in front of you and bring awareness to how you feel in that moment.

When we are fully anchored in presence, we are free of the

past, the future, and the well-rehearsed narrative we have running through our mind. Thoughts of the future or memories of the past aren't real in the moment: They are just thoughts. Mindfulness is the practice of becoming aware of when we are lost in the trance of the mind and then consciously and deliberately bringing our awareness—our mind and body—back to the reality of the present moment. This is something we can practice throughout the day and in every single experience.

I remember one of my first "penny-dropping" mindfulness moments, when I was waiting in line at a post office. I was near the back of a long, barely moving queue, fidgeting and huffing. I was so irritated with the inconvenience. My mind was also elsewhere, worrying about my dog who I had left in the car, parked in a short-stay loading bay outside. It was a chilly autumnal day, so he was very safe, but I knew he hated being left on his own. I felt the sensation of anxiety rising in my chest, but instead of being consumed by it I could hold the feeling in my awareness. In doing so, I realized it was my thoughts that were creating my uncomfortable experience of that moment. The irritated, stressed-out, impatient headspace I was in wasn't going to make the queue go any quicker. It wasn't going to stop me getting a parking ticket, or make a difference to how my dog was feeling in the car. I realized I was creating my own experience and anxiety through my thoughts, judgments, and resistance to what was, after all, just a post-office queue. In that realization it was almost as if a bubble burst. I stood there in exactly the same physical reality, but my experience of it was completely different. I felt lighter and empowered with an overwhelming sense of clarity and peace. In awareness I realized I had a choice—I could leave the queue and move the car or come back another time. Or I could remain in the queue and be patient, practice mindfulness, and be with what was actually there in that moment.

Being present in the moment—which includes being with our thoughts, feelings, and emotions—is something that requires a fluid practice of non-judgmental awareness and compassion. You don't need to find time to practice or do anything differently, necessarily, but instead remember to notice when you've got lost in thought, then forgive yourself and consciously bring your awareness back to the reality of what is: the present moment.

We can't control anything in this life other than our own response to it. Through a dedicated mindfulness practice, we can shift from reacting to responding, and create a much more peaceful and empowering reality for ourselves in the process.

Where did mindfulness come from?

Mindfulness is a widely accepted and adopted practice for health and well-being across the Western world today, despite having been often dismissed as "woo-woo" nonsense decades before. The West's appetite for mindfulness began slowly during the 1980s and 1990s due to the secularization of the practice, paired with the increasing amount of scientific evidence to back up its validity. By the mid 2000s, mindfulness had become a recognized and established approach to managing stress and anxiety and to enabling a more balanced state of well-being. This growth in interest paved the way for a multibillion-dollar industry to establish itself, which Data Bridge Market Research predicts to grow to $9 billion by 2027 in the United States alone.

The lineage of mindfulness dates back thousands of years to ancient spiritual, religious, and mystical teachings, often associated with Buddhism and Hinduism. Despite these age-old roots, today the practice somehow feels more relevant than ever before in Western society, where levels of stress, anxiety, and suicide rates are increasing year on year.

The practitioners Jon Kabat-Zinn, Herbert Benson, and Thich Nhat Hanh have each contributed greatly to the popularization of the modern mindfulness movement, including—most impressively—its integration into modern medicine. An overwhelming amount of research confirms that mindfulness offers a number of benefits for mental, emotional, and physical well-being. These include increased attention span, reduced levels of stress, anxiety, and depression, improved sleep quality, pain management, a strengthened immune system, an increased volume of gray matter in the brain (the area responsible for regulation of emotion) and, even, assistance with weight loss.

What actually is mindfulness?

like to think of my mindfulness practice as the clicking of fingers to snap me out of being lost in a daydream of thought. I see it as a signpost pointing me back home, to embody a state of open, loving presence—and to really be here now. Jon Kabat-Zinn, often nicknamed the "godfather" of modern mindfulness and arguably the most influential person to integrate the practice into modern medicine, describes mindfulness as "paying attention in a particular way, on purpose, in the present moment, and non-judgementally." To be mindful is simple in theory but, as most of us will know, it is often trickier to consistently embody throughout our everyday, busy, complicated lives—especially in the face of complex challenges. Over the last ten years as a journalist—of curiously exploring, practicing, and facilitating meditation guidance—my understanding, definition, and own personal practice have changed greatly, and I have come to accept with excitement that this is a lifelong assignment.

I often hear people say they can't practice meditation or mindfulness because their mind is too busy. What they might not realize is that by claiming: "I have a busy mind," they are, in some way, already practicing mindfulness! To know that your mind is busy requires a certain level of self-awareness, which is the beginning of a mindfulness practice.

Mindfulness guides us to gently ask: "Which part of me knows my mind is busy and which part is the busy mind?" Getting lost in thought, or being consumed by emotion, is very human. Our complex, thinking minds and our intuitive, responsive bodies—and the relationship between the two—are both the miracle of and challenge for our species.

A mindfulness practice helps us shift from living in an automated, trance-like state, consumed by thoughts and emotions, to a fully present, open state of being. It encourages us to notice when we are in a trance of the mind, to let go and anchor the mind and body back into the vast expanse of the present moment. It doesn't matter how lost we might get in the foggy trance, or for how long—the power is in awareness, and the present moment is always there, waiting patiently for our return.

With practice, we start to understand that we are not our thoughts or emotions. They are something we experience—just energy moving through our body that affects how we see the world, how we project ourselves or judge our experience, and how we feel in the moment—which, in turn, creates and shapes our "reality." For me, this idea that "thoughts are not who we are, they are something we experience" shifted from being a frustrating and irritating thing to hear, to being one of the most relieving, freeing, and exciting revelations I've had in my adult life.

To "become aware" is to have woken up from the mind's trance. It creates space between thought and reactions, and can break the hold thoughts, feelings, or judgments have over our experiences. So, really be here for a moment—right here—this book in your hand, the space you are in, how your body feels and how you feel. Anchor in, even just for a second, to the reality of this moment without attaching thought or judgment to it.

In every moment of awareness, we are offered a choice: grasp hold of thoughts and make them true, or let go, snap out of them, return to the reality of every fluid, unfolding moment. In awareness, we can then make a conscious, responsible choice— just as I experienced in that post-office queue. But, my goodness, it's not easy, and that is why I believe mindfulness is a courageous act. It requires us to take loving responsibility and to be radically honest with ourselves and others.

I see every moment of awareness as a new beginning, a fresh start, almost as if the slate has been wiped clean. It is where we are offered agency and opportunity; we can rewrite our story, heal, start to make changes, and choose love for ourselves and the planet. It starts right here, in this moment, with you.

Mindfulness requires courage

Mindfulness helps us bring what is unconscious into conscious awareness—"bringing it above the line," as Tara Brach puts it in her book *Radical Compassion*. The "conscious mind" refers to the part of our mind, and experience of living, that we are consciously aware of: our thoughts, feelings, senses, and sensations. It is our awareness of self and environment. It is the part of the mind that is responsible for short-term memory, logic, and analysis. But this only accounts for roughly 10 percent of our brain activity, the remaining 90 percent is "subconscious"—therefore outside our conscious awareness. This is illustrated perfectly by many psychotherapists through the metaphor of an iceberg. The tip that you see above water is our conscious mind. Bobbing along the surface of the water are our emotions and values— experienced consciously or unconsciously. The bulk of the iceberg is submerged under water and out of view. This represents our subconscious mind—where self-image, beliefs, fears, habits, judgments, creativity, imagination, and projections are held. Then, right down in the murky depths is where trauma, guilt, and shame reside. This is why, for some, the body is considered to be the unconscious mind—it remembers, stores, feels, and protects through our nervous systems what the conscious mind processes. Mindfulness—the practice of being present in the moment, with what is—helps us build a relationship of self-trust and self-awareness, befriending our nervous system and enabling us to start to understand, love, and heal our holistic self. This in itself can be both freeing and challenging. It is uncomfortable and confronting to face our truth at times, because we are facing our shadows as well as our light. It means sitting with feelings, emotions, or experiences that we might wish weren't there, but which are shaping our experience of life whether we face them or not.

It can be disheartening for people to realize that when they come to practice mindfulness and meditation, they find their problems, anxiety, stress, or depression still waiting for them there in the quiet. It can be disappointing for people to realize mindfulness isn't a shortcut to "make you happy." Instead, it makes you aware.

I like to imagine feelings and truths as little bubbles, which rise up from my core, provoked by emotional triggers, environment, thoughts, hormones, bodily sensations, stillness— or for no reason at all. Some are fun, light, and fizzy, and make me feel high and giddy. Some taste a little sour on the way up, and some are bitterly painful. What so often happens when a painful bubble surfaces is we think: "oh no, I don't want to feel that," and so we push it back down where it might fester, only to explode one day in a volcano of anxiety or turn into a heavy, weighted knot of depression.

That said, some emotions and experiences might be too hard for us to process on our own, which is when support from trained therapists, counselors or coaches is essential, especially when pairing mindfulness with trauma or addiction.

Regularly practicing the habit of bringing your awareness to the present moment (mindfulness), throughout your day and in all experiences, offers you a strong foundation to remain present at times of challenge, rather than being totally consumed by what's going on in your head (thoughts) or body (feelings). This is why mindfulness requires courage.

Mindfulness is not a quick fix

Mindfulness and meditation are disciplines that require practice, something those of us conditioned by the fast-paced, quick-fix culture in the West find hard to swallow. You can't practice mindfulness once and expect your whole physiology, neural pathways, or emotional conditioning to have changed in an instant. Mindfulness is a lifelong practice, just like brushing your teeth twice a day: You don't brush your teeth just once and find they're clean forever.

A plethora of scientific evidence proves the physiological, psychological, and emotional effects of a mindfulness practice, including the decades of research carried out by Herbert Benson through the Benson-Henry Institute. His work has proved that mindfulness increases activity in the prefrontal cortex, the part of the brain responsible for rational thinking, emotional awareness, and control. It reduces activity in the amygdala—responsible for states of fear and anxiety—while a meditation practice has been shown to increase activity in the insula, responsible for visceral feelings, instinct, and intuitive responses. Benson refers to the state of deep meditation, yoga, or prayer as "the relaxation response," and in this state he claims we "produce immediate changes in the expression of genes involved in immune function, energy metabolism and insulin secretion." Each of these benefits isn't experienced overnight or after one meditation session, and so we simply have to show up to practice.

Mindfulness is "to become familiar with"

In June 2019, the *Guardian* website published a "long read" article with the clickbait-worthy title "The Mindfulness Conspiracy." It passionately outlined the author's beliefs surrounding everything that is wrong and harmful about mindfulness. My interpretation of the argument was that mindfulness promotes a society of "snowflakes," who close their eyes to injustice and global issues. The article convincingly claimed that the passive nature of mindfulness is damaging for activism and revolution, and discourages people from standing up for what really matters. Reading it made me reflect: If my interpretation was the same as that author's, I too would have the same passionate aversion to mindfulness as he did. But my interpretation and experience of it is vastly different.

My belief is that mindfulness is not about passive ignorance or teaching people to roll over and let others walk all over them. Nor

"Acceptance is about being honest with ourselves and others."

does it mean passively watching our neighbors getting trampled on either. Acceptance is about being honest with ourselves and others; setting and upholding boundaries; and always being open to learning. It's about being where we are, feeling all we feel, making conscious choices, and taking conscious action. Mindfulness and meditation lead to increased self-awareness and, therefore, a greater sense of confidence to speak our truth and stand up for what we believe in.

I really like a phrase Dr Joe Dispenza used in a podcast interview with Lewis Howes, when asked what meditation meant to him: "Meditation is to become familiar with." To practice mindfulness is to become familiar with our senses and with the sights, sounds, tastes, touches, and smells of each moment. It is to become familiar with "self": in touch with our thoughts, feelings, and our nervous system's reactions, which all affect how we experience life. It is to become familiar with our habits, of mind and body, with what we are choosing, consciously or unconsciously. It is to become familiar with the energy that moves through us and the ecosystem that we are a part of, not separate from. It is to become familiar with the miracle, gift, and impermanence of life itself.

For me, this is a lifelong practice of remembering, slipping back into a trance, and remembering again—or waking back up. It is knowing that forgetting is part of the process—in awareness we can choose again. Catherine Franklin, a wonderful participant in an online course I offer called Discover Meditation, put it beautifully: "I've realized that mindfulness and acceptance aren't passive but are in fact the first step to change and action."

Despite the secularization of mindfulness and mounds of scientific evidence that pile up around it, it seems obvious to me that the practice eventually leads us back to spirituality. When we become "familiar with" we can see clearly. When we see clearly, we can choose wisely and deliberately. When we choose wisely and deliberately, we live more consciously. When we live more consciously, we are concerned about the greater "we," not just "me." When we are concerned with whatever is greater than us and understand that we are but one thread in a much larger tapestry of life, we can begin to experience connection and purpose. When we experience connection and purpose, we start to understand the non-dual nature of all things.

How to practice mindfulness

I think it's important to remember that to be "present"—a state of being that the practice of mindfulness returns us to—is the most simple and basic human state, which happens all by itself quite naturally, often without conscious practice. Have you ever been moved to tears by a sunset, or fallen completely in love with soft light moving through autumn leaves, or felt connected to something much greater than you when floating on the surface of the ocean, making love, singing, or dancing? Imagine if that sense of presence, awe, bliss, and wonder was how you lived each day, in every moment. I see a mindfulness practice as the gateway to consciousness, and the simplest way to start practicing mindfulness is to really use your senses.

Take a deep breath down to your belly, and bring your awareness to your eyes. Notice what is here, in this moment, surrounding you—the light, subtle movements, textures:

- Bring your awareness to your nose and notice any subtle scent or smell carried in the air.
- Really pay attention to the sounds around you, including the silent space between the sounds.
- Notice how your whole body feels—are there any areas of tension that you can consciously soften? The mind–body connection is undeniable, so listen to your body's physical cues. Tight shoulders, a clenched jaw, or a gripping tummy show us what's going on in our mind.
- Notice where your mind is—what thoughts, stories, judgments, or narratives are running.
- Think about how you feel in your heart. Place a hand over your heart and ask yourself: "How do I feel right now?"

This practice could be carried out when you are sitting in your car stuck in a traffic jam, in the shower, or in a post-office queue. In my own experience, this simple, understated practice has been life-changing.

What is mindful eating?

Mindful eating, or conscious eating, is quite simply just one means of practicing mindfulness, no different from any other. The principles of mindful eating can be applied to any activity you might like to pop the word "mindful" in front of: creativity, movement, art, conversation, gardening, love-making, jigsaw-building, arguing—you name it! But having a specific focus to your practice, such as food, can start to embed new and healthier habits, while helping you understand yourself a little better. When we fully embody the practice in one focused area, we can then more easily apply it to other areas of life.

Mindful eating doesn't just relate to the mindful consumption of food—how you prepare it and how it tastes—it goes a lot deeper than that. It involves noticing the emotional state you are in when you reach for and consume food. It is to listen to your body and take stock of how you feel during and after eating. It means offering your awareness and consideration to where the food you choose has come from and how it was grown and produced. It's about waking up to and lovingly investigating your habits and choices, which weave throughout all aspects of life, not just your relationship with food. It is an opportunity to live and embody your values.

Mindful eating doesn't require you to learn anything new or to become an expert in nutrition. It doesn't restrict, condemn, or vilify any food that you or others choose, nor is it a reason to preach, advise, or prescribe what you should or shouldn't be eating. Instead, it is a practice of gentle curiosity, non-judgmental awareness, conscious choice, and a joyful celebration of food. It is about bringing your full, focused attention to your relationship with food, without judgment. That clarity then informs and empowers conscious choices in the future.

Food is pleasure and a sensual experience. We eat with our eyes; we are lured in by the smell and we often make audible sounds when we take a mouthful of something delicious. The smell of certain foods can evoke emotion and memories. The practice of mindful eating asks us to deliberately tap into our senses and pause to notice the colors, textures, and presentation of each meal. It is to smell the food before it is consumed and to really taste it.

Becoming curious about how and what we eat can be used as a tool for self-care, self-awareness, and connection. Even the simplest meal can come loaded with energy, stories, culture, and tradition. Sharing food is a means of bringing communities together: A meal can unite lovers, families, and strangers, and has done so within all cultures for centuries.

Food isn't just fuel to keep these miraculous human bodies of ours functioning efficiently: It represents an intimate relationship between us and the earth. The food we eat has an effect on our bodies and minds and, in turn, the choices we make have an effect on the planet and the producers, growers, and communities who enable it. What you eat and how you eat could be seen as a declaration and embodiment of your subconscious values, and your relationship to yourself. Food is a source of pleasure; it is knowledge, life, and love. Food is just great, isn't it?

To practice mindful eating is to ask important questions:

- What benefit would eating this food have for my body?
- Where has the food come from?
- Who or what might have been impacted or involved in the journey from its origin to the plate?
- What nutrients is this food giving me?
- Why am I reaching for this food?
- How do I feel right now?
- Am I thirsty?
- Is this a nutritional craving or an attempt to alleviate mental or emotional unease?
- How does it taste/smell/look?

With these simple considerations and a more conscious awareness, a shift will naturally occur in the ethics of the food you buy and consume.

Start your mindful eating practice right where you are

If you've ever been wine-tasting, you will be familiar with the mindful approach to the experience. First, you study the wine visually, to notice the colors and textures. Next, you smell the wine to become aware of its subtle aromas. Then you taste the tiniest sip and become curious about flavors and how they change on your palate. And, finally, you kick back and savor your glass of wine. What if we applied this same mindful approach to our first coffee every morning, or our dessert? To do so would be to practice being present and mindful while also letting ourselves savor, celebrate, and truly enjoy our food.

Any change in life requires one thing—for us to take that first step in a new direction. So, start right here, in this very moment, exactly as you are:

- Pause and be present before every meal or hot drink; be still or seated and notice how you feel.
- Smell the aroma and notice what happens to your taste buds.
- Notice how hungry (or thirsty) you really are and how you feel in your body.
- Notice the colors and textures, and how the meal or drink looks.
- Offer a sense of genuine gratitude, even if silently in your mind, for what you are about to consume.
- Really taste the first mouthful, making sure you take your time to chew and notice the changing flavors.
- Avoid multitasking while you're eating: Be present with your meal and company.
- Stop eating when you are full.

CHAPTER TWO

FOOD AND SELF-AWARENESS

When we take the time to pay attention to our relationship with food, we can start to understand ourselves a little deeper, and become more self-aware. By observing our own behavior, with kindness, we begin to notice our unconscious habits or emotional reactions—what we might call operating on "automatic pilot."

Emotional eating

The term "emotional eating" describes when people use food to manage, cope with, or distract from their feelings. I call this my "reach-for" food. You surely know the state: When you're feeling upset, stressed, bored, lonely, or lost in the trance of the mind, it is the food or drink that you reach for, unconsciously, to soothe you—maybe realizing later that, somehow, the whole package, bowl, or bottle has gone.

Within the context of mindful eating, we are going to shift the focus from *what* it is we are reaching for to *why* we might be reaching for it, and what emotional state we are in when we do. Putting the "comfort food" itself at the center of the equation only distracts us from what actually has the power to make a change: you. So, for now, let's not worry too much about what your "reach-for" food is, whether it's a chocolate bar, a big bag of chips, a family pack of some sugary snack, or a glass of wine. Instead, let's get curious about when, how, and why we reach for those things.

That said, some "reach-for" foods or drinks are clearly more harmful than others. If you realize, on consideration, that you might have a harmful or unmanagable addiction, awareness—or facing it—is an empowering and critical moment to ask for help.

I remember vividly the first time I consciously watched myself "reach for" food for comfort. I was in my early thirties and I had just found out that a group of friends had met up for a pub lunch just minutes from my house, but had forgotten to invite me to join them. This came on top of some work stress and an argument with a family member and, in that moment, I was triggered. When I personally feel triggered—when an external stimulant challenges my ego's sense of self, resulting in the engagement of the body's sympathetic nervous system, or the fight/flight/freeze response— my usual reaction is to flee. No fighting or freezing for me when I'm in the trance of the mind. No, it's avoidance all the way. I turn and run for the hills.

In that situation, I unthinkingly grabbed my keys, got in my car, and just started driving. I had no idea where I was heading, just so long as it was as far away from my feelings as I could get. The petrol light in my car came on, so I was forced to stop and fill up with fuel. While I was waiting in line to pay, I reached for a giant bar of chocolate. Then I paused in awareness, my hand in mid-air. Right there—I was "reaching for." I had been consumed by the trance of my mind and emotions and I was reaching for chocolate to be my comforter, to act as a numbing agent in search of relief.

My hand hovered for a moment or two in clarity. "Ooh, how interesting," I thought to myself—swiftly followed by "Why not?" I bought the chocolate and started to shovel it into my mouth as soon as I got back in the car, without even tasting it. But that time, it was different. Through awareness, I had somehow reclaimed my power. I continued to watch myself as I ate the chocolate in one go, as the well-rehearsed pattern played out. Next, I noticed the rising feeling of guilt for having eaten a giant bar of chocolate in one go, which would result in feeling even more rotten about myself. I still felt those things on that occasion, but almost as if I was watching it all play out, rather than being consumed by it.

"For all of us, one thing I feel certain about is that non-judgmental awareness and self-compassion are the first steps toward change."

Chocolate has always been my "reach-for" food. I know now that when I am centered, emotionally stable and present, a large bar of chocolate can easily sit in my pantry and be savored, bit by bit, as a treat. But I also know that when I am in an unconscious frame of mind, the whole bar will be consumed within seconds and without me tasting a bite.

The reaction most of us have—reaching for food or drink to soothe or comfort us when we feel stressed, anxious, or consumed by thought or emotion—is nothing to feel guilty about. Some psychologists argue it is subconscious conditioning, from when we were babies and our cries were instantly soothed by milk. I do find tumbler-like takeout and reusable cups interesting—I can't help but compare the suited army of city workers rushing through town slurping on their coffee cups with a child cradling a tumbler to soothe itself.

Emotional eating could indicate an inability to process emotions; it could show how we feel about ourselves and our level of self-love. It could reflect the degree to which we are present in each moment of our everyday lives or it could be the result of an unconscious habit. In more extreme situations, emotional eating has been linked to a form of self-abuse and chronic low self-worth and can result in eating disorders, either over- or undereating. If you identify with this, you are not alone, and I strongly encourage you to seek help or guidance from a therapist or expert (the website beateatingdisorders.org.uk is a useful place to start).

For all of us, one thing I feel certain about is that non-judgmental awareness and self-compassion are the first steps toward change. So, how do you become aware of your "reach-for" foods? You can start by simply getting into the habit of practicing a conscious pause (like pulling the car over) before you consume anything. Remember to breathe, consider what's really going on for you in that moment, and notice how you feel. Instead of food being the enemy, or the answer, mindful eating suggests you shift your focus to investigating what your body needs, uncovering for yourself what healthy, nutritious, loving food choices might be. Food can then become your medicine or an opportunity for pleasure.

Mindful eating can be pretty simple: a practice of non-judgmental, deliberate, conscious awareness followed by choosing something nourishing, delicious, and aligned to what's right for you. Take a moment to reflect on the following questions:

- What are your "reach-for" foods?
- What emotional state do you associate with this action?
- What are the triggers for this emotional state? Meditate on this closely to uncover the core of the trigger, not just what's on the surface.
- If someone else was experiencing this emotion, what would you say to them?

Eating habits

Forming any new habit and embodying a mindfulness practice takes time. Even with the best of intentions, most of us easily forget and slip effortlessly back into old, well-worn ways.

A study published in the journal *Appetite* suggests that "habit is one of the most powerful predictors of eating behavior." Our habitual behaviors, patterns and choices usually happen without conscious awareness: automated behavior performed as an energy-saving mechanism which, in itself, is extremely helpful for us humans. It means we don't have to relearn skills, knowledge, and everyday tasks over and over again. It is just that some behaviors and habits are clearly more beneficial than others. Little information is needed to make a habitual choice and habits are often intrinsically linked to external or situational cues. What, how, and when we eat is often a result of habit, not conscious choice.

What do you eat for breakfast, and why? Is it well considered and nutritionally balanced, or is it mostly out of unconscious habit? When it reaches 9 p.m., do you have a habit of reaching for a glass of wine or something sweet? Do you consciously prepare and mindfully consume snacks and check in to ask yourself: Am I really hungry? Am I just thirsty? What does my body need as opposed to what do I want? Or do you snack unconsciously?

In his article "How Long Does it Actually Take to Form a New Habit?," James Clear notes that: "On average, it takes more than two months before a new behaviour becomes automatic—66 days to be exact. And how long it takes a new habit to form can vary widely depending on the behaviour, the person, and the circumstance." However, research on the length of time it takes to change a habit varies extensively. One study by students at

University College London, published in the *European Journal of Social Psychology*, claimed that in order for a habit to become automatic, it requires anywhere from as little as 18 days to nearly a year, depending on the habit itself, the environment, and the individual. So, as with all things, it is a personal process, and it takes time.

Changing a habit is complex and not just about willpower—it can also be physiological. For example, habits that are formed based on pleasure create the chemical dopamine, which leads us to craving it again and cements the habit further. Habits can be situational: I arrive at work and make a coffee, or I smoke a cigarette after dinner, or I get together with Claire and I drink a gin and tonic. Habits can also form as a result of our own sense of self-worth but, arguably, for a habit to be a habit, it has to be automated. Awareness is one of the most potent tools for conscious choice and change.

Form an intention to be more conscious of your food choices and eating habits, and maybe keep a journal to record any insights you have. Keep a note of how you feel physically and mentally before, during, and after consuming, and even when purchasing food. Set reminders or display visual cues to prompt awareness—stick notes on your refrigerator or pantry doors, for example—and forgive yourself when you "forget." See any awareness practice, even if infrequent to begin with, as a genuine positive; perpetuate that positive feeling and reward yourself every time you choose wisely, rather than dwelling and berating yourself if you slip up—because, who doesn't? Keep small promises to yourself, start where you are, and make micro-changes, rather than building a daunting mountain to climb.

Intuitive eating

Mindful eating promotes the idea of intuitive eating: to be attuned to eating when we are hungry and stopping when we are full. It is to pay non-judgmental awareness to our cravings and to savor and enjoy every bite.

Cravings are an interesting topic because there are differences to be understood in what drives a craving—is it physiological, emotional, situational? When we practice mindful eating we are present in our body and ask ourselves: How hungry am I? Am I full? How do I feel emotionally and physically?

Mindful eating leads us to become intuitive to the body's needs. Strange cravings in pregnancy, for example, are claimed by some scientists to be innate wisdom in the body to guide the expectant mother to consume the nutrient she needs, such as sodium or calcium. When I started choosing a mainly plant-based diet, I was paying more attention to what *not* to put on my plate than seeking a balanced diet from what I did. After a while, I found I started to crave protein and iron—not meat itself, but I intuitively knew what my body needed, something that had changed. I consciously upped my plant-based protein and iron intake by adding more garbanzos, spinach, broccoli, and tofu to my diet, and it did the trick.

Cravings could be seen as physical cues from the body to maintain optimal health when we consider them from an intuitive sense, but we know the opposite is also true: Food itself can cause cravings. So, what about those pesky little cravings that aren't so nutritious? Have you ever noticed that the more junk food you eat, the more you crave? Have you ever wondered why this is? Food cravings are linked to the region of the brain responsible for pleasure, reward, and memory. A hormonal imbalance or imbalanced microbiome (gut bacteria) may be a cause and, as

"Generally, mindfulness helps us to recognize and manage stress, to process our emotions in healthier, more conscious ways, and it improves sleep."

we've discussed, emotions play a major role too. For example, stress has been connected to an increase in cravings for sugar and sweet foods in women. Avoiding becoming hungry, ensuring you drink the recommended eight glasses of water a day, and getting a good night's sleep have all been linked to reducing food cravings. Generally, mindfulness helps us to recognize and manage stress, to process our emotions in healthier, more conscious ways, and it also improves sleep.

Mindful eating can help us start to recognize whether a craving is intuitive or addictive. First, it helps prevent cravings to start with, as the practice encourages us to eat when we are hungry, stop when we're full, and recognize and honor our body's cues. It promotes the act of chewing and eating more slowly, which, in turn, aids digestion. Most importantly, the practice asks us to be present when eating, consciously checking in with our physical and emotional state, and thinking about what nutrients are in the food we are reaching for. If there is little or no nutritional value in what you are craving, ask yourself: Is this craving being driven by habit, emotion, or my glorious taste buds? Another really powerful question to ask is: What would this craving satisfy?

When you are craving food emotionally, it is often one specific food that you're obsessing about—such as ice cream or cake—rather than a need for nutrients (iron, protein, or sustenance of some kind). There might be a sense of aimlessly searching (wandering around your kitchen in a trance) or habitually reaching for food, rather than a conscious choosing. Maybe it's not long since you finished your previous meal.

When you are truly hungry and have a desire to eat—eat! But some time should have passed since your last meal, and it's better if it is something that will benefit you nutritionally, not just your taste buds. Tune into your body and notice the physical cues it gives you for your next meal: Your tummy might feel empty or maybe you sense a slight slump in energy. When you do eat something—chewing properly, taking your time, and really enjoying what you are consuming—you should feel fully satisfied afterward.

Here are some playful ways to become aware of our eating habits and start to initiate change.

Reframe what a treat is

I have found that reframing what a treat is has been unbelievably helpful in changing habits when it comes to my own food choices.

Why is it only unhealthy, nutrient-poor foods that we label a treat? A treat for what? More often than not it is a treat for our taste buds alone—not for our gut microbiome, our energy levels, our skin, our clarity of mind, or even the planet. I wonder whether our subconscious understanding of what a treat is might be different if we were "treated" to raspberries every Saturday as children, rather than candies. The definition of a "treat" is something we have every once in a while, because we enjoy it. A treat isn't something you have daily, or even several times a day—that's a habit.

When you eat mindfully—which is to bring all your senses to the experience of eating—a simple piece of fruit can taste like an exquisite delicacy. A berry picked straight from the bush is a gift from the earth: a treat. (The dessert recipes in this book are largely sugar free, dairy free, and gluten free, yet I guarantee they will still taste like a treat.)

Call food what it is

People often have a resistance to calling the things they eat exactly what they are. A conscious attempt at remaining unconscious, maybe? But a fun little game you can play to be really conscious of what you're eating—and to start to ask yourself if this is the best choice for you—is to call the foods you consume exactly what they are. A dear friend, France, who is a huge advocate for daily celery juice, says she often calls out to her husband playfully, "I'm just going to drink my nutrients."

A bowl of home-cooked tomato soup is, essentially, cooked tomatoes. A candy bar is sugar. An apple is a sweet gift from a tree. Milk is the "teat milk" from a cow. A ham sandwich is processed pig flesh. Even calling out a cup of coffee (which I love) as a "cup of caffeine" somehow makes me more conscious of my consumption and aware of my addiction.

Realign your choices with your values

Is the food you consume aligned with your core values? How do you want to live your life and how do you want to feel?

Maybe you just want to be happy, healthy, and less stressed and to enjoy life. Maybe you want to be kind and a force for good in the world. Maybe you want to live a balanced life, to go with the flow and live simply. Maybe community and nature are important to you. Maybe you want to just say yes to life and have more fun.

Mindful eating gives us full permission to eat whatever food we want, without limits, but there is an important and critical element to a true mindful eating practice, and that is to choose consciously. Having permission to surrender any rules and restrictions around the food we eat doesn't mean it would be in

"Mindful eating is to ensure there is balance and that our values are aligned with the food we choose and consume."

our best interest, or the planet's, to scoff mindlessly, consuming junk food, cake, and all the processed food we like. Mindful eating is to ensure there is balance and that our values are aligned with the food we choose and consume.

In the UK, the boycott of plastic straws was a movement that caught on quickly and effectively. Cafés, restaurants, and bars that still serve plastic straws in drinks are very much frowned on in today's culture, in which making eco-friendly choices has become somewhat trendy. Why do you abstain from using a plastic straw? What moral judgment or conscious choice are you making when you choose a paper straw over a plastic one? Are you upholding that same value in other areas of your relationship with food, drink, and consumption? Are you as considered when it comes to packaged versus unwrapped food, the carbon footprint of what you buy or where it has come from?

Where your attention goes, your energy flows

Bring your awareness to your hands for one moment—just become aware of them. Can you feel an aliveness, a tingling sensation in the hands, just by taking your awareness there? Quite literally, "Where your attention goes, your energy flows"—a saying attributed to the coach and author Tony Robbins but affirmed by many. This not only holds true for our sensations and experiences, but it may also apply to external things in life, including the food we eat.

When we go on a diet and try to follow a list of restrictive rules—quibbling over calories, logging every item, or checking what we must not eat—we tend to think about food constantly, usually whatever we are not allowing ourselves to have. When we say, "Right, that's it, I'm not eating cake for x amount of time," all we can then think about is cake. We count down the days until our self-imposed time restriction is up and we can gorge on cake once again, only to wonder why we then feel so terrible and put any weight we've lost straight back on.

Cake isn't the problem: Cake is just cake. It is you—the consumer—who can consciously choose how much cake to eat, and how often; to mindfully notice what drives you to want it and how it makes you feel. Be empowered and compassionate with yourself as you become more curious, and know you can always choose again.

CHAPTER THREE

FOOD AND HEALTH

You are probably familiar with the phrase "You are what you eat," and know from your own experience that what you eat has an effect on your physical body. But how does the food we eat affect our mind and mental health? Being mindful of the food we consume is a widely publicized aspect of well-being, and rightly so. The food we eat affects our weight, mood, energy levels, gut health, physical vitality, cognitive function, and mental health. According to a comprehensive review published by *European Neuropsychopharmacology Journal*: "Accumulating data suggests that diet and nutrition are not only critical for human physiology and body composition, but also have significant effects on mood and mental well-being."

Yet, for so long, the mainstream narrative about food has focused on dieting and weight loss, driven by a society obsessed with body image. This collective fixation is fed by a multibillion-pound industry, which is reliant on people associating weight loss with self-worth and happiness, and, in many ways, seeing food as the enemy.

We are constantly bombarded with fads and conflicting advice from corporate organizations, who offer weight-loss solutions by counting calories or controlling diet. This approach often deters dieters from consuming natural foods such as nuts, avocados, and coconut oil because of their fat content, yet promotes the consumption of the corporation's own processed meals and snack bars, all with the sole aim of losing weight.

For me, this fixation on weight tends to perpetuate the notion that "when I lose weight I'll be happy/more attractive/loved, and then I will be able to accept myself." But what so often happens in this race for weight loss is that the finishing line seems constantly just out of reach. Dieters become obsessed with counting calories and feel inadequate on the journey toward their goal weight,

"Mindful eating isn't so much about dictating what we should be eating or how we should look as about bringing awareness to our relationship with food and understanding that what we eat affects us and our wider ecosystem."

rather than focusing on feeling vibrant, healthy, and balanced within themselves.

Reaching for processed, packaged foods under the impression that anything labeled "lowfat," "no fat," or "diet" is good for you is so misleading. Such products often have little to no nutritional value, are laden with sugar, and even perpetuate the problem. According to an academic paper by Cora J. Wilen, despite a booming $40 billion diet industry in the United States, 95 percent of dieters there regain their lost weight within one to five years.

Curiously, most books about mindful eating also seem to focus on weight and body image. For me, this is a narrow view of what mindful eating encompasses. Mindful eating isn't so much about dictating what we should be eating or how we should look as about bringing awareness to our relationship with food and understanding that what we eat affects us and our wider ecosystem. It is about shifting our perspective to accept, love, celebrate, and nourish our bodies, minds, *and* the planet—and to honor that symbiotic relationship.

It seems to me that this popular approach to eating, with its fixation on "dieting," is back to front and upside down. Has this focus on weight loss compromised the general health and well-being of dieters? And for what sustainable long-term gain? A common outcome of eating natural, healthy, nutritious foods, alongside movement of some kind, is that we feel better within ourselves—mentally and physically—and we have more energy to live fully. Our weight and body shape are then a by-product of our individuality and our own unique holistic wellness, not the starting point for it. What feels right and good for you as an individual, might not be the same for me. Honoring and celebrating the differences in our body shape and size is empowering. Self-love and acceptance is a mindset, not a physical manifestation.

A beautiful friend of mine, Lisa Allen, recently shared on a retreat how she had been nurturing her own sense of worth using affirmations, mirror work, meditation, and journaling. She began to cultivate the habit of ensuring that, every time she looked in the mirror, she would compliment her beauty rather than criticizing every line or curve. She told us how she looked at her thighs one day and said to her husband, "It's so strange, they haven't changed in shape or size, but they just look so much better: In fact, they look great!"

Body image, and indeed our whole relationship with food, is deeply personal and unique, and can be highly sensitive. A mindfulness practice of any kind helps us to find our center, to notice with compassion and curiosity when we feel triggered and to remember that we are exactly who, what, and where we are meant to be. I wish you knew how beautiful you really are, as you are.

Food and mental health

The food we put into our bodies can either aid cellular repair and give us energy or it can drain us of it. For example, processed grains (white bread, white pasta) are energy drainers due to the fact that the nutritious bran layer is stripped away in their production. When we consume processed grains, we experience a sharp rise in blood sugar and insulin levels, followed by a sharp drop in energy. Whole grains, on the other hand, are more nutritionally complete and allow for a slow release in energy.

Junk food, fast food, and processed food, which many in Western cultures seem to crave, provide very few nutrients and tend to be high in saturated fat and low in fiber. Eating them can slow digestion, leaving us feeling sluggish, over-full, and then hungry again very quickly. Low-calorie foods, promoted by the diet industry as snacks and meal substitutions, have been linked to hormonal imbalances and increased cravings, and have a slowing effect on the metabolism.

Years ago, I took part in a fundraising campaign called "Live Below the Line," run by the charity The Hunger Project. Participants could only spend £1 a day on food, for five days. If a pinch of salt was added to food, it had to be included in the budget. If I used a handful of herbs I'd grown myself, I would have to factor in the cost of the seeds, container, and production. For breakfast, lunch, and dinner—and all beverages other than tap water (which you are reminded is still a luxury for a lot of people in the twenty-first century)—I had to spend no more than £5 for the duration of the challenge.

I bought oatmeal (75p), which I mixed with water, and some bananas (69p) for my breakfast and as a snack. I bought some cheap packet soups (£1) for lunch, along with a big bag of pasta

"The mind itself has an effect on our ability to digest food too."

(£1), a bag of frozen mixed vegetables (£1), and a small pot of (reduced) pasta sauce with the leftover change for my dinners. By the end of day two I felt unsatisfied and cranky. By day five I felt sluggish, unhealthy, and in a severely low, unmotivated mood. When the challenge was done I bought every variety of fruit you could imagine and topped it with coconut yogurt, chia seeds, flax seeds, and a drizzle of honey. I drank a liter of orange juice and mindfully gulped a large oat latte and, oh my goodness, it all never tasted so good.

Taking part in the challenge changed the way I thought about food in many ways. I was struck by how atrocious I felt having eaten the same stodgy, mostly processed, foods with low nutritional and high sugar content, even after just five days. It hit like a blow to the gut that eating this way is the only option for many people living on the poverty line in the UK.

I was struck by the drastic effect the food I ate had on my experience of life: my ability to concentrate and apply myself to my work, the energy and enthusiasm I had to exercise, and my motivation to do anything at all. Consequently, I became acutely aware of my privilege being able to choose to eat healthily.

Food poverty is a devastating issue that is inexcusable in this day and age. The inability to afford or have access to healthy food results in a wide range of negative impacts on individual health and wellness, in the short and long term. Organizations such as The Trussell Trust in the UK and Feeding America in the United States are working tirelessly to combat food insecurity and, although we won't dive deeper into this important issue here, I urge you to educate yourself on this issue and support organizations where you can.

My experience of living below the poverty line for just 5 short days, not only startled me into recognizing my own privilege, it also made me experience the drastic effect poor nutrition had on my mind, energy levels, and experience of life.

The mind itself has an effect on our ability to digest food too. Stress is claimed to deplete vitamins essential to energy production and regulation of the nervous system, so it could be argued that the link between food and stress, or low mood, becomes a self-fulfilling prophecy. We're stressed or depressed, and so we reach for junk food with very little nutritional value, which makes us feel worse—and around the cycle goes.

Research indicates that, for some, improving diet also helps improve symptoms of depression. The results of one clinical trial, published in *BMC Medicine*, showed that eating fresh fruit and whole grains, and limiting the amount of processed, sugary foods, had a significant effect on symptoms in people reporting moderate to severe levels of depression.

Numerous studies link food intake to conditions such as heart disease, cancer, diabetes, Alzheimer's, and dementia. A diet made up mainly of saturated fats and refined sugars, with low fruit, vegetable, and water intake, has negative effects on cognitive ability, while a balanced, nutrient-rich and varied diet is essential for brain function. According to the National Institutes of Health: "Having too much sugar, salt or fat in your diet can raise your risk for certain diseases. Healthy eating can lower your risk for heart disease, stroke, diabetes and other health conditions."

Opting to eat healthily, if we can, is, then, better for our bodies, minds, and the planet, while considering how "healthy food" has been grown and produced is just as important.

Hell no, GMO

Pesticides, hormones, and antibiotics are widely used in animal and plant farming to increase and modify supply and quality, but the effect these chemicals have on our health and the environment is alarming.

Mindful eating is to remember that your food has been on its own health journey. The cod you order deep-fried in batter on a Friday night may very well have ingested microplastics, which can transfer from the gut of the fish to its flesh, meaning that you too are consuming plastic. The hormones and antibiotics pumped into cows will be carried through to their milk and flesh, so you may be consuming those chemicals in your tea or wedged between a bun. While there is surprisingly little publicized research into the effects of GMOs (Genetically Modified Organisms) on human health, the pesticides and herbicides used in crop production have been linked to birth defects and non-Hodgkin lymphoma, and are potentially carcinogenic according to the World Health Organization.

Meanwhile, the effects of GMOs on the environment are deeply unsettling. In the United States, the decline of monarch butterfly populations by 90 percent in the last 20 years has been linked directly to the increased use of a herbicide that kills common milkweed, a flowering plant the butterflies require for breeding. GMOs affect ecosystems and biodiversity, and can result in contamination, with serious economic, ecological, health, and social consequences.

Being aware of how the food you eat has been grown is an essential consideration in a mindful eating practice. As defined by the UK Government's Department for Environment, Food & Rural Affairs (DEFRA), "Organic food is the product of a farming system which avoids the use of man-made fertilizers, pesticides,

"Mindful eating is to remember that your food has been on its own health journey."

━━━━━━━━━━━━━━━━━━━━━━━━━━━━━━━━━━

growth regulators and livestock feed additives. Irradiation and the use of … GMOs or products produced from or by GMOs are generally prohibited by organic legislation." For food to be labeled "organic," at least 95 percent of its ingredients must come from organically produced plants or animals.

Organic food is, arguably, better for individual and environmental health because, well, it's natural. But, as always, there are counter-arguments that suggest organic farming or eating organic food are no better for us than using GMOs. An essay on the NHS website cites "no strong evidence to support the health benefits from eating organic instead of conventional foods," going on to say: "Obviously there are some other reasons, besides nutrition, that may make people choose organic food, such as concern for the environment." This reads to me as if "concern for the environment" is a cute intention to have, and I found it curious that the author uses the word "conventional" for genetically modified foods—are they suggesting that naturally grown foods are the unconventional ones?

Mindful eating is about choosing consciously for your own individual health, but also being aware of how those choices affect the health of others: the bees, the soil, the air quality, producers, and the environment.

Consciously purchasing the food we buy, or "voting with our wallets" as some call it, sends a message to the profit-hungry industries that hold the puppet strings. It tells them what we care about and want as consumers. An article published in the *Guardian* in February 2020 stated that, in 2019, UK sales of organic food and drink had risen by 4.5 percent, reaching a record high of £2.45 billion. A follow-up article, published later that year, claimed that sales of organic products had increased further in the UK during the first coronavirus lockdown. I was fascinated and deeply encouraged by this trend, especially at the pivotal moment in our collective experiences represented by the pandemic.

Gut health

Have you ever noticed the number of sayings about intuition and extreme emotion that reference the gut? "Trust your gut"; "It takes guts to do what you did"; "Spill your guts"; "What he said felt like a punch to the gut"; "I had butterflies in my tummy." We feel strong emotions—nerves, anxiety, love—in our tummies. We have always known that our gut, in some way, is an important silent navigation system, where truth can be found.

The gut has been called the second brain, and for good reason. Over 100 million nerve cells are found along its lining, famously the same number of cells as in a cat's brain! These cells are responsible for communicating directly to the brain via the vagus nerve and neural pathways, which are connected to our emotional state.

The physiology of gut health is concerned with maintaining a balanced microbiome in the gastrointestinal tract, which has been linked to immune support, weight management, and general digestive health. Conditions thought to be associated with a gut microbiome that is out of balance include autoimmune disease, diabetes, low mood, and depression.

The coronavirus pandemic seemed to have made consumers more concerned with preventative health support, particularly for the immune system. In the UK, buying trends before and during the resulting lockdowns saw a sharp rise in the purchase of non-dairy, organic foods, and probiotic products.

Mindful eating can help support your gut health in many ways. First, it encourages you to eat more slowly and to remember to chew, which, as we'll see later, can aid digestion. According to Michael Mosley, presenter of the BBC Four show *Guts*: "When we eat, it normally takes 20 minutes for food to get from the stomach to the ileum, causing the release of [the gut hormone] PYY and the message to the brain, 'I'm full.' That is why it is better to eat slowly, to give the stomach a chance to tell the brain you have had enough before you overeat."

A mindful eating practice also reminds us to consider the quality and balance of the foods we are eating; to choose a range of colorful, organic vegetables, fruit, whole grains, legumes, and beans and limit the amount of sugar and processed foods. Experts in gut health also encourage us to consume fermented foods such as kimchi, sauerkraut, and kefir.

Food and healing

Health and healing are holistic and individual; all things don't work independently from one another and there is no one approach that fits all when it comes to our personal health. It's a jigsaw puzzle made up of: the food we eat; the water we drink; how often we move our bodies; the information we feed our mind; the company we keep; the

"My brush with cancer made me put the brakes on and reassess. I was reminded to surrender, on a cellular and spiritual level."

environment we live in; the air we breathe; our relationship with our nervous system. All of these contribute to our general health, our potential, and our ability to thrive.

Good health isn't just about eating nutritious food. While giving conscious consideration to the food and chemicals we put in or on our bodies is vital to our health and well-being, it is also important to acknowledge the bigger holistic picture.

In the summer of 2019, I was diagnosed with stage 1 cervical cancer, much to the shock and disbelief of many people around me. If I had a pound for every time I heard someone say, "I can't believe you got cancer, you eat so healthily/you meditate/you eat mostly vegan/you do yoga/you don't drink alcohol," I would be a very wealthy lady. The experience was a huge shock to me, too, and it provoked me to reflect and reconsider my approach to health and healing. I was very lucky that it was caught at such an early stage, and I personally found so many answers to the questions I was asking myself by studying the work of Dr Gabor Maté. Healthy food was important, but it made up only one slice of the health-and-healing pie for me. Rather than finding my own healing in a green smoothie or 75 rounds of sun salutations every morning, I found it in surrender and intuition.

I realized that, up to that point, I had been trying so hard to build, accumulate, and achieve in life, it wouldn't have mattered how much kale I ate, or whether I obsessed over only eating "healthy foods," because other areas of my life were out of alignment. My brush with cancer made me put the brakes on and reassess. I was reminded to surrender, on a cellular and spiritual level.

I realized my own health, healing, and happiness didn't hinge on restricting myself or feeling guilty about my past decisions or mistakes; what mattered were my choices and mindset in the "now." I realized that I live each day more brightly, fully, and with more zest for life when I eat well. For me, healthy food choices are consciously made because I genuinely want to uphold them: Those choices help me live my life with more energy. I am no longer reluctantly dragging myself to healthy foods, like I might have done when I "dieted" in the past. I am not choosing healthier foods out of fear, or as an insurance against disease, or in search of my self-worth, but, rather, because those choices truly help me to live better today, while I am alive.

Making conscious food choices isn't a stand-alone solution to good health and healing, but it is one vital element that cannot be ignored, especially when considering the much broader picture of individual, societal, and planetary health. The miraculous body that holds you—a body that enables you to explore the world, experience pleasure, create, work, and feel—requires love, fuel, rest, nutrients, vitamins, and minerals in order to thrive. Remember that you have agency over what you put in and on your beautiful body and the ways in which you nourish and nurture it.

CHAPTER FOUR

SEEING FOOD AS SACRED

see food as an opportunity for self-care—in terms not only of the quality of the food I choose to put in my body but also the intentional ritual performed around eating it. In my own journey toward self-love and acceptance, I noticed how my relationship with food was intrinsically linked to the power that lies in making and eating that food—in making it sacred.

After reading Louise Hay's book *You Can Heal Your Life*, I found myself repeating the affirmation: *I love myself, therefore I feed my body delicious, nutritious, wholesome food*. But, despite this promise to myself, my relationship with food wasn't always so loving.

When I was younger my relationship with food was dysfunctional, and only as an adult have I realized that I used to suffer from an eating disorder. My teenage years were fraught with challenges and my way of coping was to eat very little. I'd feel a sense of accomplishment when I'd make it to the end of the school day having only eaten one chocolate bar, or to bedtime having only had one hot chocolate, which I would usually make myself throw back up. I didn't do it to be skinny—I hid my skinniness under baggy jumpers. I did it, I realized later in life, because of my own chronic sense of low self-worth and an unconscious search for control.

Much later in life, I found myself newly single in my early thirties, and a lot of my daily habits and routines changed. I noticed that one drastic difference when living alone was how I ate. If I was cooking for friends, or a date, I would buy the best ingredients, spend time preparing the meal with great care, and present it with flair and creativity. I would lay the table, light a candle and we would eat at the table. But I would never go to that much trouble, or in fact any trouble, when I was eating by myself.

I wasn't surprised to find multiple studies claiming that eating alone is associated with a number of health risks, including poorer diet, weight gain, and making unhealthy choices. Much of the research on this topic suggests a bias toward the conclusion that eating with other people is better for our health. However, I believe there is something much more powerful to be realized. In my new single life, often eating by myself, I stumbled across a powerful mindset shift in the direction of self-love and responsibility.

One night, sitting on the sofa, stirring a bowl of cereal with questionably in-date milk as "dinner," I thought to myself, "Wow! Is this how much I value myself?". I reflected for a while and wondered: If I truly loved and cared for myself, why wouldn't I feed myself with the same love and nourishment as I do others? If I were feeding my inner child right now, would I feed that creative little girl a sour bowl of mush?

I made a promise to myself, right there and then that I would feed myself as the guest of honor in my own life. I would cook for myself as if Zac Efron were coming over or I was feeding a whole family that I adored. I decided to make the commitment to nourish myself as if I loved myself and considered myself a person worthy of nourishment.

I still uphold that promise to this day. Don't get me wrong— every now and again I have an oven pizza, something quick and easy, or a Thai takeaway. But mostly I cook for myself as I would for someone I truly loved: home-cooked meals, made with love and presented beautifully.

To make something sacred means to set it apart from unconscious habitual actions or reactions. To make food sacred is to consider what we eat as something special and precious, worthy of gratitude and worship, just as your body deserves nourishment and care, exactly as it is in this very moment.

Mealtime rituals and traditions in the West have largely been lost in the secularization of modern culture. For example, the Christian custom of saying grace before every meal, with the whole family together around the table, has been replaced with convenience meals, eaten separately or in front of the television. That simple, beautiful ritual of pausing before a meal to say thank you—to the earth, the food, or the energy of life for making it all possible—is a simple practice that can help us eat more mindfully.

Imagine if you paused before every meal, simply, even just silently in your own being, to say thank you. Imagine if you took a moment to notice the food in front of you, became aware of its fragrance, colors, and textures. Imagine if you considered, just for a moment, the journey the food had been on to make it onto your plate, and then whispered a sincere thank you before you start eating. How would that feel?

The importance of eating as a family or community will be explored in the next chapter but, for now, appreciate the food you eat as a sacred gift from the earth and remember the simple, lost art of gratitude and ritual at mealtimes, because they can change everything, including our relationship with food. Say thank you, light a candle, be present, be curious, go slower, savor the process, and taste every bite. Make the food you eat and the ritual you create around it sacred.

Keep chewing

What I haven't yet admitted is that, without conscious practice, I am quite possibly the most naturally unmindful person! This is why I think very simple mindfulness and self-care practices have had such an incredible impact on my life. When I worked in busy office jobs, I would often eat lunch at my desk,

"Eating can become habitual and unconscious, to the extent that we often barely taste the food we eat, let alone really enjoy it."

not taking my eyes off the computer screen. I'd shovel a sandwich into my mouth and wash it down with a slurp of coffee while typing, reading, rushing. I was rarely ever present with the food I was eating, and still now need to check myself to slow down and be present.

Eating can become habitual and unconscious, to the extent that we often barely taste the food we eat, let alone really enjoy it. You might be eating your favorite meal in the world and not really taste it because your attention is on Netflix, your work, or lost in the dream of thought. When we're not present with the food we eat, more often than not we don't chew nearly enough as we're eating it. Chewing affects our gut health, and a lack of chewing gives us a poor indication of when we feel full, or even whether we feel satisfied.

The saliva produced when you chew starts to break down your food right at the start of the digestive process. As the swallowed particles of food move along the gut, water and essential nutrients are absorbed. Chewing properly means we eat a little slower too, which itself has been linked to weight management, because the brain needs a bit of time to register that you have eaten and when you are full. The nutrients absorbed by the gut also stimulate hormones that regulate hunger. Eating slowly and chewing will not only help digestion but also allow time for flavors to be released, meaning you can really taste and enjoy your food.

I was pretty shocked to find out quite how much we should be chewing—it is an incredible amount. Ayurveda, the ancient Eastern approach to medicine and lifestyle, suggests we should chew our food 30 times before swallowing, while a research study published in *The American Journal of Clinical Nutrition* asked participants to chew over 40 times, resulting in participants feeling less hungry and more satisfied having eaten less.

Personally, I think let's not get too hung up on counting every mouthful, creating yet more rules to follow, restricting ourselves in other subtle ways when it comes to food. Instead, do it once— chew a mouthful of food 35 times and notice quite how much chewing that really is! And then, simply adopt a mindful eating practice: Go a little slower, be present, chew more, notice the changing flavors, and enjoy the pleasure of each and every bite.

Cooking is alchemy

Cooking is alchemy, creativity, and play. For me it's about tasting, testing, experimenting, and creating. All hail Jamie Oliver and his approach and ethos toward cooking, recipes, and food. He tends to suggest we "add a dollop of this" or "a splash of that," directions that inspire me to have some fun.

I'm not a professionally trained chef but, my goodness, do I love to cook. I have put my heart into creating bowls of deliciousness for retreat guests over the years, but my real love of cooking started many years ago when I worked as a support chef in a hotel restaurant.

The manager, whom I nicknamed Uncle Peter, was a wonderful, trusted, fatherly figure for me while I worked there. He would plate something up beautifully, precisely swirling a *jus* onto a plate and placing a leaf here or a sprig there. Then he'd set me to work, recreating plate after plate of colorful food art. I loved it.

Uncle Peter taught me how to use a knife properly, what efficiency looks like in practice, and how to chop an onion with symmetrical precision. He taught me to really care about the way food is presented and that music and good vibes in the kitchen make for better-tasting food. I don't know where Uncle Peter is these days, or whether he still listens to Shania Twain on full volume while he cooks. I don't even know if he would remember me. But I do know that the joy I find in creating food art on a plate is mostly thanks to his guidance.

Every meal you make, every sandwich, every bowl of fruit you assemble is a creative act. The extent to which you engage in the creative process is up to you and the time you have to play, whether you make it a simple sketch—chopped fruit in a bowl drizzled with coconut cream—or a masterpiece—a three-course banquet fit for a queen.

Most simple home-cooking recipes—especially the plant-based ones you'll find in this book—aren't intended to be followed to every inch or crumb. Home cooking is not the same as making complicated gourmet meals, where measurements need to be followed precisely in order for the food to rise or set. You can adjust all the bowl dishes in this book as you go and you are encouraged to do so: adding a bit more of one flavor, simmering for longer to thicken, or switching an ingredient for whatever needs using up. Even once you've served up a meal, you can still adjust it by adding seasoning or herbs. See these and any home-cooking recipes as a template from which you can be creative and play, not as a regimented set of rules.

Cooking intentionally

The "vibrational energy" of food is an essential consideration in Ayurveda, which claims that the closer the food is to its natural, living organic state, the higher its energetic vibration. If we eat "living" foods, we absorb those high vibrations. "High vibration" foods essentially mean foods that are real, living, and nourishing, that add nutrients to or help detoxify the body.

Energy goes both ways. It is a symbiotic relationship between the energy we receive and the energy we give. Have you ever eaten a meal and just known that it's been made with love?

I once cooked for the book launch of a dear friend and mentor, Maggie Kay. Her book, *Diving for Pearls*, was about her own journey of self-discovery and finding love. While I cooked, I played my favorite love songs loudly, belting along, wooden spoon in hand. I reflected on romance and the magic of falling in love while I stirred and tended to an enormous pan simmering with tagine.

The tagine was a hit among the book launch attendees, and I was gobsmacked when a quiet, intuitive, graceful woman came up afterward and said, "That meal was so heart-warming and wholesome. Thank you. I could almost taste the love that had been poured into it." Can our energy, emotions, and thoughts really have an effect on the meals we prepare? A researcher and healer in Japan believes just that.

Dr Masaru Emoto, author of *The Hidden Messages in Water*, claims that our intentions, words, and how we feel—our energy—can change the physical world around us. His research first focused on water. In controlled conditions, a large group of participants was asked to direct positive energy, words, emotions, compliments, and prayers toward samples of water, while other samples had negativity, threats, and insults directed toward them. His results showed that the molecular structure of the water that had received loving intentions had changed to appear under a microscope as beautiful, geometric structures, almost like a mandala shape; whereas negative energy and emotions changed the molecular structure of the water to appear chaotic, incoherent, and scattered.

He then experimented with rice under similar conditions. He divided portions of rice into two separate containers and asked schoolchildren to direct kind words and wishes toward one container, and to bully and insult the other. After 30 days, the rice that had been complimented appeared fresh and unchanged, whereas the bullied rice had gone rotten with mold.

In Yogic philosophy, it is widely accepted that energy and emotion are present in animals, too, and that they fear death, just like us; all living beings have an innate desire to live. So, when an animal is brought into a slaughterhouse, it is in a heightened state of fear: The whites of its eyes show, it is restless and full of anxiety. Its body floods with hormones released from the endocrine glands (prompting a fight-or-flight response), which then infuse the tissue of the animal. The theory suggests, then, that meat-eaters are in turn ingesting the animal's fear, anxiety, and stress.

Thoughts, words, and even actions are energy. Emoto's research suggests that energy is not only transferred from the food we eat to us, but also transferred by us to food as we prepare and eat it. But his research also suggests that our whole physicality could be affected by the energy of our thoughts, since our human bodies are mostly made up of water. Maybe Louise Hay knew this intuitively when she said: "Be conscious of your eating. It's like paying attention to our thoughts. We can learn to pay attention to our bodies and the signals we get when we eat in different ways."

"I try to uphold a ritual of intention before cooking every evening meal. I will often light a candle, much as I do before a meditation, and blow it out once I've finished."

Setting an intention is an easy way to initiate a pause before cooking and eating, and to shift your energy in a mindful way. Or maybe you might like to set a wider intention for your relationship with food. This could be "to eat more healthily" or "to have more energy" or "to see food as an opportunity for nourishment." Then pause and ask yourself: Are the ingredients or meal in front of you going to help your intention come to life?

Setting an intention is to actively point yourself in the right direction. It can help you stay positive, aligned, accountable, and present. I try to uphold a ritual of intention before cooking every evening meal. I will often light a candle, much as I do before a meditation, and blow it out once I've finished. I play music, sing or dance, or listen to podcasts. Whether it does actually make the food taste any better, you'd have to be the judge, but what I do know is I find great enjoyment and pleasure out of cooking this way—and that, maybe, is all that matters.

See cooking and eating as an opportunity for creativity, positivity, love, play, and connection. Turn the music up loud just as Uncle Peter would because, as it turns out, good vibes in the kitchen might just be a real thing.

Making food sacred

The food we eat represents an intimate relationship with the planet; it's an exchange in which the earth provides and we consume. How we consume and the choices we make have an effect on the earth. Being considerate, compassionate, and intentional is an important part of mindful eating: mindset matters. Here are some simple ways to foster an intentional mindset:

- Choose "living," organic, "high-vibration" plant-based foods.
- Set an intention before cooking or eating.
- Say thank you.
- Chew, take your time, and avoid multitasking when you are eating.
- See food as a practice of self-care and feed yourself as the guest of honor in your own life.
- Honor the creative act of cooking and have some fun.
- See your relationship with food as a sacred exchange with the earth.

CHAPTER FIVE

THE JOURNEY OF FOOD

Mindful eating on an individual level involves curiosity, awareness, and agency. But this mindset also extends much wider to consider the bigger picture. A mindful eating practice might help you pause to consider: What journey has this food been on to get to my bowl? How was it produced? And who or what has been impacted and affected in its production?

Take the banana. It is a cheap, easily accessible, staple part of most British diets (and smoothie-bowl recipes), yet its abundance nowadays is somewhat taken for granted, and its political history is rarely considered. Mass consumption of anything doesn't come without a cost.

Banana plants originate from the Malaysian and Indonesian jungles of South East Asia, and were exported to China, Africa, and the Caribbean—tropical climates in which the plant thrives—by European colonists in the fourteenth century. The fruit was introduced to Britain in 1633 as an exotic and expensive luxury item, and, in the nineteenth century, banana plantations became a vital and tainted part of the slave trade.

There are over 1,000 varieties of banana, and, interestingly, they don't grow on trees, as is often assumed, but rather from a plant, making the banana a fruiting herb. According to Banana Link, an organization that works to ensure fair production and trade within sustainable social, environmental, and economic means: "Bananas are one of the most consumed and cheapest fruits worldwide: they are the most traded fruit and the fifth most-traded agricultural product. The global export value of the banana trade was estimated to be US$8 billion in 2016, with a retail value between $20 and 25 billion."

The report continues: "Bananas are also emblematic of the growing power of supermarkets along global supply chains

"What journey has this food been on to get to my bowl?"

and of the wide range of injustices present in international trade today, including unacceptable working and living conditions for many who grow and harvest the bananas, the suppression of independent trade unions and an unfair sharing of profits along the chain."

Growing bananas to meet international demand requires mass clearing of jungle. It often involves excessive use of pesticides—which not only damage ecosystems but also contaminate soil and water supplies for local communities with devastating effects—and is a labor-intensive, time-consuming process. The banana industry is dominated by a small number of cost-cutting multinational corporations, who are in many ways themselves being controlled by profit-hungry supermarkets, all held together in a web of unfair trading practices.

The history and journey of one banana, something you may take for granted as you slice it over your breakfast cereal, is vitally important to consider as a conscious consumer. Paying attention to the where, how, and who of the food we consume is mindful eating.

Alongside the benefits to your health and the environment, choosing organic food is a means of supporting the health and welfare of the growers' communities too. Choosing Fairtrade brands is one simple decision made by you, the consumer, that can have a significant impact on the health and livelihoods of those involved in production. Choosing produce that is

"Feeling a genuine, deep sense of gratitude for the food we do get to enjoy means it will taste all the better."

certified by the Rainforest Alliance is a way of considering and supporting sustainability—environmentally, socially, and economically. Choosing local, where we can, will help reduce the environmental impact of transportation. Growing your own is a meditative act of mindful living. Either way, conscious consumption lets the food industry know what is important to us as consumers.

It is often argued that organic and Fairtrade products tend to be more expensive, creating a barrier to purchase. Let's skip back to when we discussed the reframing of what a "treat" is. Expanding our awareness from "treating" our taste buds alone to the bigger picture—shifting our consideration from "me" to the global "we"—morphs and changes our definition of a treat, too. With this in mind, might we realize what a privilege it is to be able to eat a banana every day if we choose? When we consider how far that one piece of fruit has traveled, who and what is involved in its journey, maybe we might start to see the banana as the exotic sweet treat it is.

This is not about feeling guilty about the range of options available to us, but, rather, about waking up to take responsibility and ensuring our actions and choices are aligned with our values. Feeling a genuine, deep sense of gratitude for the food we do get to enjoy means it will taste all the better.

As we saw in chapter 2, our unconscious habits often start before we even make a purchase. We now realize that they continue, trance-like, throughout our whole relationship with food: shopping, preparing, consuming, disposing of waste, and packaging are all carried out on automatic pilot while our minds are busy elsewhere. As the saying goes, "Life is what happens while you are busy making other plans." When we are not present, we miss the pleasure of eating, the joy of food and the sense of alignment gained in purchasing with both your values and your taste buds.

Moving with and honoring the earth's natural cycles becomes a living mindfulness practice. We understand that we are part of nature's tapestry, not its master. Everything in our conscious reality comes from the earth and returns to it. When we abuse the earth, the environment, and others as a result of our choices, wants, and actions, we are abusing and harming ourselves— there is no separation.

Some talk of "saving the planet" as a heroic act, suggesting that nature is a commodity we own and are ourselves able to save or take care of, like a pet. In my humble opinion, the only way to win is to realize our symbiotic relationship with all things. Conscious living is to surrender to and move with the world that sustains us, not to dominate or manipulate it for our gain only.

Consciousness is the birth of responsibility, yet this can be misinterpreted as entailing separation and ownership. The responsibility of consciousness is loving choice and considered action. The small, simple choices we make as individuals in our everyday lives are what is important. Responsibility means the extent to which we move within the rhythms and cycle of our environment, and the love and kindness we show to all living beings. Mother Earth will go on, with or without us. But, while we are here, mindful living and eating are about consciously considering how gently we tread and how willing we are to give as well as take. In waking up to the privilege of our existence, we can see clearly and feel in awe of the miracle that is: the water we drink; the pleasure and purpose of the food we consume; and the impact that our choices have on everything.

Mindful eating is considering the life cycle of food

When I was a student, I worked in a bar. One of the first jobs on my shift was to chop an obscene number of lemons into even, thin slices, ready to put in drinks throughout the night. As I chopped, I would ponder each lemon, imagining the tree planted as a seed. I would wonder where it was planted, and by whom. I'd think about how it was nourished, the tree harvested, and the fruit transported. I'd imagine the lemon in a crate of thousands of other lemons, making its way by multiple means of transport from its place of origin to find its way into my hand. As I sliced, I would wonder whose drink it would end up in, only to be thrown into the bin and sent to landfill at the end of the night. That lemon had come from the earth, then gone on a wild adventure, only to return to it.

I didn't know I was reflecting on a mindful eating practice at that time, but, in many ways, that is exactly what I was doing. What we consume isn't just about us as an individual; we are not separate from the ecosystem as a whole. Everything we choose and consume involves another, and eventually finds its way back to the earth.

The cycle, as I humbly see it, goes like this: Weaved within it, and not separate from it, is the health of the individual, the community, and the environment, while another thread weaved intrinsically through the system is that of economic health, cultural trends and habits, and capitalist wealth.

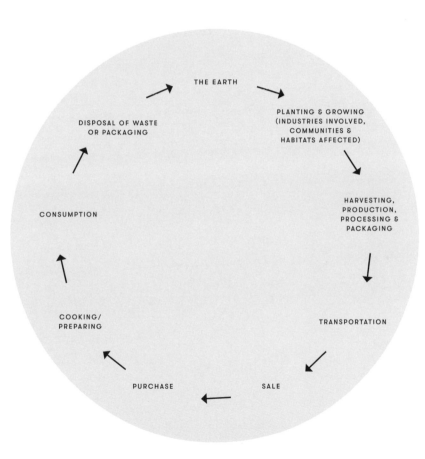

THE EARTH

PLANTING & GROWING
(INDUSTRIES INVOLVED,
COMMUNITIES &
HABITATS AFFECTED)

HARVESTING,
PRODUCTION,
PROCESSING &
PACKAGING

TRANSPORTATION

SALE

PURCHASE

COOKING/
PREPARING

CONSUMPTION

DISPOSAL OF WASTE
OR PACKAGING

"Mindful eating in itself doesn't dictate what we eat. The practice doesn't state that you have to be vegan, never eat sugar, follow a certain set of rules, or place a fence around your beliefs and ideals."

Mindful or conscious eating is about expanding our view to realize we are not separate from the whole or exempt from the problem. It isn't just awareness alone that makes a difference, but also agency and responsibility, essential components of any mindfulness practice. It is the making of conscious choices, aligned with our deepest values, that is in the greatest interest of the sustainable health and well-being of all.

Mindful eating in itself doesn't dictate what we eat. The practice doesn't state that you have to be vegan, never eat sugar, follow a certain set of rules, or place a fence around your beliefs and ideals. Instead, it asks us to wake up and make considered and conscious choices that are kind, loving, and beneficial to our bodies, minds, communities, and planet. To truly practice mindful eating, we understand we must "be the change."

The ritual of mealtimes

The act of gathering to eat together creates a meeting space for connection, where we can bond, listen, and share stories, truths, and energy. Making sacred time to come together around a table with an assortment of edible delights is a unifying tool for intentional living— an opportunity to pause, reflect, and (literally) digest. History is full of evidence for the importance of feasting, food-related celebration, and eating rituals within families, communities, and cultures. Archeological evidence indicates that the practice of communal eating and feasting was part of daily life at the time of early agricultural production, while large family mealtime scenes remain synonymous with Italian and Indian cultures, to name just two examples.

Some argue that, historically, community or family eating was largely down to convenience; cooking in bulk for a group saves resources by requiring less produce to feed more tummies, resulting in less waste. But there is plenty of evidence to suggest that the benefits of gathering around a table to eat go a lot deeper than that. Communal eating has been linked to the strengthening of social bonds and an improvement in general health and well-being. A study published in the *Global Journal of Health Science*, for example, found that sharing a meal increased a sense of happiness and social connection among participants.

This rich sense of sharing a meal has become somewhat lost in modern Western culture. Creating this sacred pause to eat and socialize is being deprioritized in just about all areas of our lives: families are less likely to eat together now than ever before; office culture promotes multitasking and eating in front of a computer without a mental, visual, or physical break; and dinner times are more likely to be taken in front of a laptop or television than at a table.

Of the many organizations I have worked for, only two had a culture where it was normal to take time away from your computer at lunch. At one, my colleague Jacqueline Gunn and I would regularly spend our lunch break together in pursuit of finding East London's finest noodles. Then, in my last job in London before moving to Cornwall to become self-employed, I would gather at lunchtime with a small group—Poppy, Sophie, Caroline, and various others—around the small table in the communal kitchen, or outside on the bank of the Thames in the summer months, with London Bridge as our backdrop. Maybe it is no coincidence that they are the people who I still keep in contact with today, many years later.

Family eating

There is significant evidence to indicate a strong link between family mealtimes and the psychological development of children and adolescents. Peer-reviewed research suggests that rarely eating together as a family leads to a higher rate of eating disorders, substance and alcohol consumption, depression, and suicidal thoughts among children and teens. On the other hand, children whose families frequently ate meals together showed an increase in self-esteem and the ability to get on well in school.

The UK-based, not-for-profit organization Bright Horizons outlines the benefits of family mealtimes on its website, including "bonding/making memories, sharing experiences, learning about each other, contributing, establishing routines, developing

"There is significant evidence to indicate a strong link between family mealtimes and the psychological development of children and adolescents."

healthy meal habits." It also offers practical tips for families on how to adopt the practice.

I only really remember those family mealtimes in the earlier years of my childhood when my family upheld the ritual of Sunday lunch. Without fail, every Sunday we would gather around the dining-room table to eat a roast dinner as an extended family. My beloved Gran-Gran would always be there, contributing some delicious culinary treat, usually Yorkshire puddings made to perfection. My Aunty Meme would join us from time to time, along with neighbors and friends of mine or my brother's from horse-riding or soccer. I remember the trifles and the wishbones. I remember finding caterpillars in the curly kale, picked fresh that morning from the local farm stand, and Mum eating one, deliberately, to prove to my brother and me that we should still eat our greens. There were disagreements and troubles as well, but among it all I remember the profound sense of comfort in ritual.

My friends Richard and Tia Tamblyn inspire me enormously as they eat as a family of five—with three young children—every day. Tia recently mentioned, in passing, how interesting it is to notice how table conversations were changing as her younger twins approached six and a half. She noted how mealtimes had shifted from just trying to get the children to all

"Gathering to eat and feast together as a wider community is an intrinsic part of human history, evident within all cultures, traditions, and religions."

eat their meals, be nice to each other, and stay at the table, to starting to be able to listen to each one and ask questions about their day.

They shared their reflections with me on why it's important to them to uphold this ritual, despite the obvious challenges:

Richard: I wish we could say we have the kids all regimented around the table. But amid mainly appalling manners and one-upmanship, there are threads of human interaction appearing! We do have all family meals together, and with whoever is here, so that the habit is hopefully formed—a bit like a meditation practice really.

Tia: For us, family mealtimes are fundamental to the rhythm of family life. We've always eaten most of our meals as a family, even when the children were very young. I've sometimes questioned this choice, given the chaos and mess that is created when three young children get stuck into a meal (at one point we had three children under two years old), but the sense of coming together and connection feels like an important juncture within the day. Sharing a meal means that we check in with each other, become part of each other's offloading and reflecting, even if that's simply hearing an argument recounted or rehearsed! At times we've included gratitude questions as a regular feature of mealtimes, although this isn't something we always do; however, we've found that bringing them in can become especially useful if the chat steers too far from a space of calm! I think the children have a broader palate having eaten most of their meals with us. I always cook one meal for everyone, albeit with adaptations such as extra chili for Richard or no mushrooms for the twins.

Our children are now 8 (Cyra) and 6 (twins Otto and Nell), and we are just starting to turn a corner, seeing insightful conversations begin to emerge at mealtimes rather than simply firefighting the chaos of spilt drinks/loo stops/disagreements. It's just wonderful when we all sink into a moment of connection about a topic someone has brought to the table. I hope that, as the children get older, these moments will increase and that, above all, the habit of mealtimes as a space where we come together, share, laugh, and learn from each other is part of their expectation of how you show up in relationships within family life.

Breaking bread

Gathering to eat and feast together as a wider community is an intrinsic part of human history, evident within all cultures, traditions, and religions. The biblical term "to break bread together" suggests the connection between food and social bonding has been strong for millennia. Just as research has demonstrated a link between family mealtimes and an increased sense of self-esteem and well-being in children and teens, similar conclusions have been made from research involving adults. The Big Lunch, an initiative pioneered by the Eden Project, the eco visitor attraction in

Cornwall, carried out a national study in the UK of the effects of social eating on well-being. Their research concluded that social eating significantly increases a feeling of satisfaction with life, and a deeper sense of community, happiness, and connection.

If we follow the bread-crumb trail of when this link between food and social well-being was formed in the human psyche, could we maybe make an assumption that it is rooted in social acceptance, tribal belonging, and security? If so, does the simple act of sharing a meal have any impact on our nervous system, an unconscious cue to reassure us that we are safe, part of a tribe, and that we belong?

Studies have shown that communal eating can help us relax and lowers participants' variable heart rate. When we consume a meal in a state of relaxation, we engage our parasympathetic nervous system, or "rest and digest" response, making an enormous number of health benefits possible. Better digestion and absorption of nutrients increases blood flow along the digestive tract, which, in turn, helps to reduce bloating and regulate a healthy weight.

Yet, as we have previously seen, there is no explicit reason why shared meals would have been more beneficial for early human communities, other than, of course, the convenience of cooking in bulk. Maybe that, in itself, is significant enough evidence to explain this innate link between eating together and well-being—our basic needs for survival were being met. During the coronavirus pandemic, the privilege of eating together freely in communal spaces whenever we wanted was not possible due to national lockdowns and social-distancing rules. The full impact on mental health as a result of lockdown isolation and restriction from participating in social rituals is yet to be researched, but for me, eating together with friends and loved ones was one of the things I missed the most, second only to hugs.

"Sharing food is a display of friendship, intimacy, and love that transcends the barriers of language or culture."

This link between food and social bonding is universal. Food can be used as the central focus of a celebration, like a birthday cake; it can offer an apology, or it can be gifted as a token of love, appreciation, or gratitude, like a beautifully wrapped box of chocolates. Lovers bond over candle-lit suppers and hospitality and kindness are embodied when we pull up an extra chair at the table for a stranger. Sharing food is a display of friendship, intimacy, and love that transcends the barriers of language or culture. It can help us to develop a mindful eating practice by creating an intentional pause in the monotony of our day, freeing up space in which we can share stories and laughter, or simply enjoy a quiet moment of reflection and togetherness.

CHAPTER SIX

FOOD AND STORYTELLING

nfused within a recipe are stories of different places, times, and people, which come bound in traditions and culture. Every single item of food that ends up in your tummy has been on its own unique journey, in terms of both geography and history. Recipes, methods, flavors and eating rituals are passed down through generations and adapted to meet the tastes and demands of modern living. Yet the rise of fast, convenient, ready-made meals, which families and communities rarely eat together, jeopardizes the storytelling element of food and cooking.

Food itself tells its own story. Spices, vegetables, types of fish or grains, and methods of cooking tell us of their cultures and origins, so much so that some claim food and recipes carry with them a spiritual and sentimental memory. The flavors and scents of cooking can sometimes act as a form of time travel, in which we are transported back to different times and places, evoking feelings and emotions in the moment.

Recently, I cooked with rhubarb, which I haven't done in years. The distinctive smell and sweet taste of my rhubarb pudding reminded me so much of my gran. The association was so fond and so strong that it provoked warm, comforting, loving tears to form in my eyes. The smell of burned toast, rather randomly, whisks me back to Wellington, New Zealand, in 2006. On my way to the little café where I worked, I would walk down a narrow lane with tall blocks of flats on either side, and every morning for three months I would be met in that lane by the smell of burned toast.

Telling stories with food has evolved in recent years through the use of social media. We photograph our breakfast, lunch, and dinner and post them to Instagram, telling the world a story of who we are, what we care about, our tastes, and our culture. In some sense, the food we eat becomes part of our identity and how we present ourselves to others.

"The flavors and scents of cooking can sometimes act as a form of time travel."

It's easier to feel part of a much bigger story when we buy food locally. One of my childhood Sunday lunch rituals would be to accompany my dad to the local butcher, Nick, to select a cut of meat from an animal that had grazed nearby farmland. When you know where the wonky carrot that you slice into a bubbling pot of warming winter soup has come from, it somehow feels more comforting and engaging. This isn't lost on companies trying to sell us their produce. Engaging in a story in some way does seem to resonate with us and influence both the way we buy and consume food and the pleasure we get from it. We feel part of the story and, therefore, emotionally invested in it, helping us to make considered choices.

The importance of honest storytelling and conscious consumerism is essential for Will Price, owner of High Steaks, a street-food vendor serving Argentinian-inspired steak sandwiches, based near Bristol. He sources his meat with three broad factors in mind: ethics, quality/taste, and price. "I want my food to taste amazing while being realistically priced for the street-food market, and I want it to have been produced in a way which respects both the planet and our bodies," he told me. He ensures that the meat he sells is pasture-fed locally, aged, free to roam, and not pumped full of antibiotics.

Will admits that it is often impossible to tell his customers a clear story about where specifically their meat has come from—which farm or exact location—due to the volume of meat he requires. "I've had to be honest with my customers and less

"Bowl food was traditionally a means of using up scraps while ensuring nutritional balance was met in times of scarcity and it provided a convenient way to consume street food."

specific. There are a lot of unscrupulous butchers and restaurants who make claims about the origin of their meat that simply can't be true." He highlights an organization called Farm Wilder, which supplies beef reared in a manner that is beneficial to the environment in many ways: "I, personally, recognize that we meat-eaters need to eat less meat overall, and my hope is that the meat we do choose will be produced using the methods that organizations like Farm Wilder endorse."

With all this in mind, storytelling is a powerful way of engaging and integrating mind, body, and emotions into our mindful eating practice. A paper written for the *Journal of Business Research* outlines three stages for linking pleasure with eating, in order to attain a sense of well-being: contemplation, connection, and creation.

Mindful eating is about contemplation—making considered, conscious choices and being with the food that is in front of us. It is about connection—between the consumer and the earth, and being mindful of the food's journey from origin to bowl. And it is about creation—cooking is creativity, alchemy, and play.

Honoring the story, tradition, and heritage of the ingredients we use and the recipes we follow is important, but to keep our relationship with food conscious and present, there must also be room for play and experimentation. If we don't pay attention to our food's story, we are not practicing mindful eating. If we eat the same things over and over again, we fall into an automated relationship with our food, just as in other areas of our lives. Being curious, testing, experimenting, bringing a beginner's mind to our experiences and rewriting the story again and again can help us choose love for our bodies and the planet, through the food we consume.

The origins of bowl food

The demand for "bowl food," a popular term used to describe nutritionally balanced meals served in one bowl, has exploded on the food scene in recent years. Maybe this is because it offers people a quick, easy, creative way of making a balanced meal. A cynic might argue that bowl food provides millennials hungry for "likes" with photogenic fodder for their social-media newsfeeds, but serving an assortment of grains, vegetables, fruit, protein, and dressing in a bowl isn't a new concept. Its heritage is steeped in culture and traditions from all four corners of the earth. So, regardless of your inclination to photograph your food, there is a lot to love about the resurgence of comforting, rich, and nutritious "one bowl" recipes.

Bowl food was traditionally a means of using up scraps while ensuring nutritional balance was met in times of scarcity and it provided a convenient way to consume street food. Eating from a bowl—as opposed to the more formal way of eating from a plate with a knife and fork—made it easy for manual workers or large families on low incomes to consume filling, wholesome, balanced meals. Today, repurposing leftovers isn't a sign of poverty or hardship, but rather one of mindful consumption and conscious,

"For me, food served in a bowl somehow just feels more comforting and wholesome."

sustainable living. In a Western society waking up to become more conscious of its health choices, yet still requiring food on the go, maybe this is where bowl food gains its crown.

Some psychologists claim that eating food out of a bowl has a psychological effect on our eating experience, because we often hold a bowl in our hands, and therefore closer to our noses. In his book *Gastrophysics*, Charles Spence playfully investigates a variety of eating quirks, including why food seems to taste better when eaten with your fingers or heavy-weighted cutlery, or whether the color of your plate itself makes a difference to our perception of taste. He suggests that, by dishing up our food into bowls, we are more likely to hold the weight of our meal in our hands, making our brains think the food is more substantial.

Bowl food is endlessly customizable. Variations can easily be made when serving up to fussy friends or family members, while the recipes themselves can be adapted by switching up which grains, vegetables, or dressing you choose by preference (or by what needs using up in the refrigerator). For me, food served in a bowl somehow just feels more comforting and wholesome. As celebrity chef Nigella Lawson says in her book *Simply Nigella*, "'Bowl-food' is simply shorthand for food that is simultaneously soothing, bolstering, undemanding and sustaining." I couldn't agree more. Bowl food is essentially a simple, nutritionally balanced, flavor-packed, filling, comforting, "one bowl" meal—what's not to love?

Traditional bowls

With a little investigation it is easy to uncover bowl food recipes from just about every country and continent around the world: from poke bowls in Hawaii, ramen bowls in Japan, and pho bowls in Vietnam, to soups and stews in Great Britain and Ireland and bibimbap bowls in Korea … the list goes on. Although the origin of the popular and trendy term "buddha bowl"—often used to describe a grain or vegetable bowl—is uncertain, assumptions have been made that it derives from the traditional way in which Buddhist monks acquire their food. Monks (who are vegetarian) wander the streets with a bowl that is filled by their neighbors and townspeople with food items, usually rice and vegetables. Here's the low-down on a few of the most popular bowl dishes from around the world:

Smoothie bowl

- Originates from: Brazil
- Traditionally consists of: blended banana and acai pulp
- Now popular in: California, Australia, Hawaii, my house
- A brief history: The most traditional smoothie bowl is the now super-trendy acai bowl. Acai pulp, which is rich in fiber and antioxidants, has always been a staple part of Amazonian people's diets. Its rise to popularity in cultures outside the rainforest is claimed to be due to Carlos Gracie, the founder of Brazilian martial art Jiu-Jitsu. Gracie advocated his own self-branded "Gracie Diet," which largely centers on maintaining a neutral pH balance in the blood. The Gracie Diet included a recipe that blended banana with frozen acai pulp, and so the smoothie bowl was born.

Poke bowl

- Originates from: Hawaii, with influences from Japan and China
- Traditionally consists of: a grain base (usually rice) and a protein (usually raw fish), topped with seaweed and sauce (typically soy sauce)
- Now popular in: North America and emerging throughout Europe
- A brief history: In Hawaiian, *poke* (pronounced po-kay) means "to cut into pieces." Traditionally and historically, it is a ceviche dish, using up scraps of fish, seaweed, and nuts. With the arrival of Chinese and Japanese immigrants, however, the dish was adapted to include rice, soy sauce, and sesame oil, which still form the basis of a poke bowl today.

Ramen bowl

- Originates from: Japan, adapted from Chinese noodles
- Traditionally consists of: soy broth, noodles, Chinese-style roasted pork, spices, bean sprouts, mushrooms
- Now popular in: worldwide
- A brief history: Post-war Japan saw the introduction of wheat flour, which was used to make noodles while rice production was compromised. Ramen bowls were a staple food in Japan in the 1950s and 1960s, and by the 1980s had become trendy, popular, and experimental. Today, ramen is a dish that is key to Japan's cultural identity.

What are the stories you tell yourself?

There is a shadow side to storytelling we must consider in our mindful eating commitment because, after all, the ego's favorite game is to tell a story.

Maybe take a moment to reflect: Have you felt resistance to anything we have discussed in this book? Have you been triggered by anything (when our ego's sense of self has been threatened)? Have you identified with something and thought to yourself "Ah, that is so me—I do/think that." Hold whatever comes up in your loving awareness, then gently encourage yourself to take responsibility and to choose again.

The ego's favorite stories, when it comes to food, might sound a little like one of these:

The "I can't/won't cook" type—I used to be one of you! I hated cooking at home, could never be bothered, and had convinced myself I couldn't do it. It's all mindset, and the beauty of mindset is it can be changed. Follow a recipe as a guide; practice, explore, and you can't go too wrong.

"I don't have time"—Do you have time to watch television or scroll through social media? Can you take 20 minutes from your screen time to home cook something simple? Can you spend time at the weekend batch-cooking ready for the week ahead? If you have children, can you involve them in the cooking process with you? Listen to a podcast, turn the music up loud, or treat cooking as a creative and reflective meditative process.

"Healthy food tastes bad/boring"—Play with flavors—spices, herbs, and seasoning are essential in plant-based cooking. We like whatever we are accustomed to, but taste does change over time. Someone who takes sugar in their tea and starts to wean themselves off it might not enjoy the tea quite as much for the first few cups, but slowly they adjust—until they can't stand any sugar in their tea at all. Be patient with yourself and know that, like everything, it just takes time.

"Healthy food is too expensive"—It doesn't have to be. If you're buying raw, fresh products rather than packaged, processed stuff you might be surprised at how little you can spend in a weekly shop, and how far a small selection of whole foods goes when you batch-cook. If you minimize the number of processed foods you add to your grocery basket, that part of your food budget is then available to buy real, whole foods. And remember, everything comes at a cost: If you're not paying for it, someone or something else will be.

Other people's judgment

As we make more conscious choices and change our habits, we may meet resistance from those around us, who are very quick to share or project their own ego's stories onto us. This might manifest itself in the form of others teasing or belittling you, or trying to convince you to stick to your old ways (often their ways). They might shout much louder about how much they love eating meat or how much wine they drink—which is just their ego's attempt to justify their own choices.

"Honoring and respecting individuality is an essential component of mindful eating, but, if you meet resistance, be mindful of what that brings up in your experience too."

I often find that the people who have the strongest reactions to what I am choosing are those who seem to lack the ability, or willingness, to change themselves. If someone's own relationship with food is balanced and healthy, they aren't really concerned about what anyone else eats or drinks. We are all trying our best and making decisions that are right, at any moment in time, for ourselves as individuals. Honoring and respecting individuality is an essential component of mindful eating, but, if you meet resistance, be mindful of what that brings up in your experience too. Try not to take it personally: Refocus on your own choices, remind yourself of your intention, and choose what is right for you. After all, you are your own best teacher and the writer of your personal story. Through mindful eating, and a wider mindfulness practice, we are simply reminded to choose love.

CHAPTER SEVEN

FOUNDATIONS AND RECIPES

Those is an old saying that goes: "Cooking is love made visible." My hope is that this saying encapsulates what we have explored through these pages—that cooking is alchemy, and eating together deepens and strengthens self, family, community, and environmental connection. It is love made visible!

By definition, "cooking" is a "practice" or a "skill." The process of cooking in itself is a playful and purposeful way to practice mindfulness; and skill comes through practice. The beauty with home cooking is, the more you practice the more knowledge and confidence you have in creating meals that you and your family will love. Be OK with making mistakes and messing up, because cooking is about play. Disastrous meals make for a great story, if nothing else, at the end of the day! The more knowledge and confidence you have, the more you are able to follow your intuition and experiment with meals.

There are some very simple foundations which form the basis for the most popular "bowl foods"—smoothie bowls, soup bowls, and buddha bowls. I share some of my own recipes for each of these types of bowls foods in the recipe section of this book but you can play with these basic foundations to create your own—using your favorite flavors and ingredients or maybe experimenting with what you have in your pantry to use up:

Smoothie bowl foundations

- Add a liquid: coconut water, alternative milks, apple juice, water
- Add a thickener: banana or oats
- Add one or more fruits (whatever you like or have in)
- Add a natural sweetener: dates, maple syrup, honey
- Add a spoonful of seeds: chia seeds, flax seeds

- Add some protein: avocado, nuts, spinach, or a dollop of nut butter
- Add a topping for crunch and texture: e.g., granola, more seeds, coconut flakes, fruit, nuts

Soup foundations

- Add the base elements: onion, garlic, oil, and spices
- Add a liquid: vegetable stock, coconut milk, miso broth, water
- Add one or more vegetables: potato, sweet potato, broccoli, carrot, corn—for example
- Add one or more herbs: cilantro, basil, rosemary, dill, tarragon
- Add a carbohydrate (optional): e.g., pasta, beans, garbanzos, lentils

Buddha bowl foundations

- Choose a grain: rice, quinoa, barley, millet
- Choose a protein: garbanzos, lentils, tofu, beans, eggs, hummus
- Choose a leaf: lettuce, spinach, arugula, kale, Swiss chard
- Choose one or two cooked vegetables: sweet potato wedges, eggplants, potatoes, parsnips
- Choose one or two raw vegetables: carrots, radishes, tomatoes, snap peas
- Choose a seed or nut: cashews, pumpkin seeds, sesame seeds, pine nuts
- Choose a dressing: satay sauce, balsamic dressing, soy sauce, hot chili sauce, vinaigrette

Stocking your pantry with a few staple items means there will always be something you can prepare as a home-cooked meal— often in just as much time as it takes to heat and serve processed foods. Being conscious of where you shop is another essential consideration in a mindful eating practice.

Big supermarkets are incredibly convenient and somewhat unavoidable in the reality of a busy life. However, I know that when I buy my vegetables from the local farm stand or a vegetable box at the end of a neighbor's gate, with an honesty box for payment, it just feels great. The lower-priced supermarkets in the UK, such as Lidl and Aldi, offer good value and often locally sourced produce, but, frustratingly, often
seem to wrap vegetables in plastic. Although, plastic wrap prolongs the shelf life of fruits and vegetables, the environmental impact of excessive plastic usage, for me, requires mindful consideration.

The Good Shopping Guide website features a ranked comparison of the ethics of each UK supermarket in relation to animal welfare, GM (genetic modification) and Fairtrade. As of March 2021, Marks & Spencer and Sainsbury's appear at the top, with Asda, Iceland, and Tesco at the very bottom. In the US, Whole Foods Market, is considered to be the most ethical grocery store, with fresh organic produce and grass-fed meats readily available, while all of Trader Joe's own branded product are sourced from non-GMO produce.

It is true that buying food from a farmers' market, a refill store or farm stand might take a little more planning, especially when living in a city, and can often seem more expensive but vegetable-box delivery services help with access issues and it is amazing how far a big box of veg can go when home cooking. Just as it is with other areas of mindful eating, it is not about condemnation or feeling guilty about our choices, but rather simply ensuring that we are making conscious decisions where and when it is possible.

The recipes in this book commonly include some the following basic items. With your pantry stocked with these, you should be able to reach for this book and make something quickly and easily at any time of day.

Pantry items

- Good-quality canned chopped tomatoes
- Canned garbanzos
- Canned coconut milk
- An assortment of dried herbs and spices
- Vegetable bouillon cubes
- Brown rice
- Rice noodles
- Rolled oats
- Mixed nuts and seeds
- Chia seeds
- Assortment of dried fruits
- Coconut oil
- Olive oil
- Sesame oil
- Soy sauce
- Honey or maple syrup
- Fresh seasonal vegetables and fruit
- Onions
- Garlic
- Alternative milks, such as oat milk

"I hope these recipes inspire you as a home cook while offering you a pleasant surprise at just how tasty it can be to cook and eat this way."

The recipes I share with you now are some of my absolute favorites to make and serve—to friends and family, as well as on retreats. Each one is extremely simple to prepare, no matter your experience of cooking. They are mostly plant-based, gluten-free, and refined-sugar-free recipes, which not only allows for wider dietary inclusivity, it also offers a basis upon which you can make these recipes your own by switching any ingredients to suit your own dietary preferences—no judgment. I hope these recipes inspire you as a home cook while offering you a pleasant surprise at just how tasty it can be to cook and eat this way.

Before you explore the recipe pages and bring the recipes to life in your own home, here is a brief recap of some of the very basic mindful eating principles we have explored.

Mindful eating 101

- Make eating sacred with ritual
- Practice gratitude
- Set an intention and be intentional about your food choices
- Be present, avoid multitasking, and eat more slowly
- Savor and enjoy the pleasure of food
- Be curious, compassionate, and forgiving with yourself as you consider your own habits and relationship to food
- Make considered conscious choices
- Choose love—for yourself, others, and the planet. Treat yourself as the guest of honor in your own life
- Choose "high vibrational," organic, natural, and real food, where possible
- Realize the symbiotic relationship between you, the food you eat, and the earth
- Play, be creative, make a mess, express yourself, have some fun
- Apply this guidance to all aspects and activities of life, not just your relationship with food!

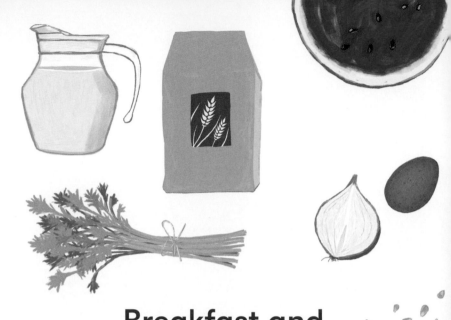

Breakfast and brunch bowls

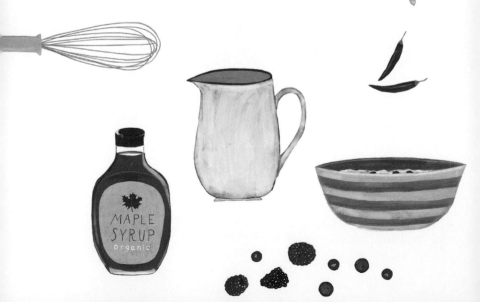

Banana, cacao, and peanut butter smoothie bowl

SERVES 2

Smoothie

1 ripe banana

1 tbsp peanut butter

1 heaping tbsp cacao powder

2 heaping tbsp gluten-free oats

1 tbsp maple syrup

2 pitted dates

1 tbsp chia seeds

scant 2½ cups oat milk or coconut milk

Topping suggestions

berries or chopped fruit of your choice

handful of natural granola (to give texture and crunch)

sprinkling of dry unsweetened coconut

sprinkling of chia seeds

drizzle of maple syrup

Method

1. Place all the smoothie ingredients in a blender and whizz until smooth. Pour the smoothie mixture into two breakfast bowls and add your choice of toppings.

2. Take some time to create a beautiful-looking bowl. Play with different colors, textures, shapes, and sizes with your toppings and take your time to sit and enjoy.

Chia seed oatmeal

SERVES 2

1 banana

2 large pitted dates

scant 1¼ cups oat milk (or your favorite alternative milk)

1 tsp ground cinnamon

1 tbsp maple syrup

4 heaping tbsp chia seeds

1 ripe mango, mashed

1 tbsp chopped mixed nuts of your choice

1 tbsp pomegranate seeds

Method

1. The night before, mix the banana, dates, milk, cinnamon, and maple syrup in a blender. Transfer the mixture to a bowl and stir in the chia seeds with a spoon. Cover or seal and place in the refrigerator overnight.

2. The next morning, divide your chilled porridge between two small bowls or glasses and spoon over the mashed mango flesh. Sprinkle chopped nuts and pomegranate seeds over the top and enjoy.

Overnight oats

SERVES 2

Oats

scant 1¼ cups gluten-free oatmeal

2 tbsp coconut yogurt (or any alternative yogurt)

scant 2½ cups oat milk or coconut milk

1 tsp chia seeds

1 tsp vanilla extract

1 tsp maple syrup

Topping suggestions

chopped mixed nuts of your choice

handful of your favorite berries,

or grated apple

drizzle of maple syrup

Method

The night before, mix the ingredients for the oats together in
a bowl with a spoon, then cover and place in the refrigerator
overnight. In the morning, give it a good stir and separate into two
small bowls. Top with a sprinkling of nuts and berries and a drizzle
of maple syrup.

Watermelon smoothie bowl

SERVES 2

Smoothie

7oz watermelon flesh

2 kiwis, skinned

1 banana

1 tbsp chia seeds

1 tbsp maple syrup

juice of ½ lime

scant 1¼ cups coconut water
(or plain water)

Topping suggestions

spoonful of granola

sprinkling of chia seeds

1 tbsp dry unsweetened coconut

any fruit of your choice

edible flowers for decoration
(optional)

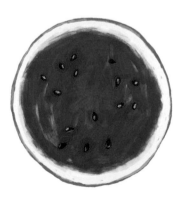

Method

Whizz all the smoothie ingredients together in a blender. Pour into two bowls and arrange the toppings decoratively around each bowl. Alternatively, for a bit of a wow factor, use the hollowed-out watermelon as the bowl.

Baked eggs

SERVES 2

1 small white onion, diced

dash of olive oil, for cooking

1 garlic clove, crushed

½ red chili, finely chopped

1 red bell pepper, sliced

14oz canned good-quality chopped tomatoes

1 tsp ras el hanout

1 vegetable bouillon cube

10 ripe cherry tomatoes (on-the-vine tomatoes have the best taste)

handful of fresh basil, chopped

salt and pepper, to season

4 eggs

Method

1. Preheat the oven to 350°F (325°F convection).

2. Sauté the onion in the oil for a couple of minutes until browning. Add the garlic, chili, and red bell pepper, and sauté for another couple of minutes. Next, add the canned tomatoes, ras el hanout, bouillon cube, and cherry tomatoes, and give everything a good stir through before reducing the heat. Simmer until the mixture starts to reduce and thicken.

3. Take off the heat, then add the basil and season with salt and pepper. Pour the tomato mix either into two small ovenproof dishes or ramekins, or one larger ovenproof pan or dish. Make a space in the middle of the mixture and break the eggs into the hole. Place in the oven to bake for 10–15 minutes until the eggs are cooked to

your preference (runny or hard yolk). Sprinkle over any remaining basil and serve with toast or bread for dipping.

Coconut oatmeal with hot stewed fruit

SERVES 2

3 heaping tbsp frozen or fresh
mixed berries
2 tbsp water
½ tsp vanilla extract
1 tbsp honey
100g gluten-free oatmeal

15fl oz coconut milk
1 tsp coconut oil
1 tbsp chia seeds
½ tsp ground cinnamon
2 tbsp maple syrup
1 tbsp coconut flakes

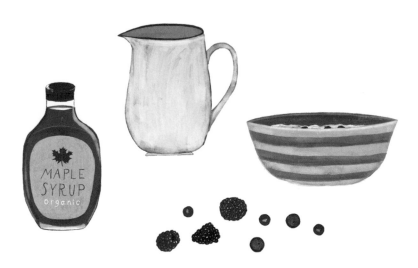

Method

1. Place the berries (either fresh or frozen) in a pan, add 2 tablespoons of water and ½ teaspoon of vanilla extract. Add the honey and squash the fruit a little with a fork. Bring to a boil, then reduce to a simmer while you prepare the oatmeal.

2. Pour the oatmeal into a pan. Add coconut milk and bring to a boil for 5 minutes, stirring continuously. Add the coconut oil, most of the chia seeds, cinnamon, and maple syrup and mix through. Pour the oatmeal into two bowls and spoon the hot berry mix over the top. Sprinkle over the remaining chia seeds and the coconut flakes, plus an extra drizzle of maple syrup.

Brunch buddha bowl

SERVES 2

8 new potatoes

1 red onion

drizzle of olive oil, for cooking

1 tsp garlic salt

4 flat mushrooms, sliced

2 garlic cloves, diced

2 handfuls of fresh spinach greens

salt and pepper, to season

1 tbsp fresh rosemary, coarsely chopped

8 cherry tomatoes, on the vine

7oz tofu (or use scrambled egg as a non-vegan alternative)

½ tsp smoked paprika

½ tsp ground turmeric

splash of alternative milk of your choice

1 ripe avocado, halved

drizzle of balsamic glaze (optional)

Method

1. Preheat the oven to 400°F (375°F convection). Cut the new potatoes into fourths and coarsely slice the red onion. Place together on a baking sheet, then coat with olive oil and sprinkle

with garlic salt before putting in the oven.

2. Meanwhile, heat a little oil in a skillet and sauté the mushrooms for 5 minutes, then add the garlic and spinach, and season to taste. Cook until the spinach has wilted and the mushrooms are slightly brown.

3. When the potatoes have been in the oven for around 10 minutes, give them a little shake and sprinkle over the rosemary. Add the cherry tomatoes to the baking sheet and drizzle with oil.

4. To make the scrambled tofu, break the tofu up into little pieces with a fork and pan-fry in a separate pan with a pinch of paprika, turmeric, and a splash of milk. Season to taste and pan-fry until the tofu is heated through.

5. Cook the potatoes and tomatoes for an additional 10 minutes, then take them out of the oven and divide between two bowls. Continue arranging the mushroom/spinach mix, scrambled tofu, and half an avocado on each plate until you are happy.

6. Drizzle with balsamic glaze for taste and decoration.

Smokey seasoned breakfast bowl

SERVES 2

Bowl
4 plump, ripe tomatoes
1 red bell pepper, seeded and halved
olive oil, for cooking
1 avocado, halved

Scrambled tofu
6oz smoked tofu
1 tsp smoked paprika

salt and pepper, to season
1 tsp coconut oil

Quinoa
3½oz quinoa
250ml water
1 vegetable bouillion cube
2 tbsp pine nuts
2 tbsp nutritional yeast

1 tbsp peri-peri seasoning

salt and pepper, to season

Serving suggestion

serve with a dollop of hummus

(see p.124)

Method

1. Preheat the oven to 350°F (325°F convection). Place the tomatoes and pepper onto a baking sheet and drizzle with olive oil, then roast in the oven for 15 minutes.

2. Cook the quinoa according to the package directions, adding the bouillon cube to the water. Meanwhile, crumble the tofu into small chunks in a bowl, then mix in the paprika and season. Heat the coconut oil in a skillet and scramble the tofu for around 5 minutes.

3. Once the quinoa is cooked, strain, and mix through the pine nuts, yeast, and seasoning. Divide the quinoa between two bowls and add the scrambled tofu, roasted tomatoes, and bell peppers and half an avocado to each. Top with a dollop of hummus.

Brunch burrito bowl

SERVES 2

1 medium baking potato, diced into cubes

olive oil, for cooking

1 large white onion, diced

2 garlic cloves, diced

1 tsp smoked paprika

1 tsp ground cumin

1 tsp cayenne pepper

½ red bell pepper, diced

8 mushrooms, sliced

2 large handfuls of fresh spinach greens

5½ oz (1 cup) canned corn, drained

14oz canned cooked black beans, drained

handful of cilantro, coarsely chopped

salt and pepper, to season

1 tbsp dairy-free yogurt or vegan
sour cream
1 avocado, halved and fanned

Serving suggestion
serve with a fried egg

Method

1. Preheat the oven to 400°F (375°F convection). Place the potato cubes onto a baking sheet, drizzle with oil and cook in the oven for around 15 minutes.

2. Add a dash of oil to the skillet and sauté the onion for 5 minutes until soft. Add the garlic, smoked paprika, cumin, and cayenne pepper and mix through. Add the red bell pepper and mushrooms to the pan and cook for another 3–4 minutes. Add the spinach, corn, and beans, and cook for another 5 minutes.

3. Once the potatoes are cooked and crispy, add them to the skillet along with the cilantro, and mix the whole mixture through, seasoning to taste.

4. Divide the mixture between two bowls. Top each bowl with a dollop of yogurt or sour cream, the fanned avocado, and, if you like, a fried egg. Sprinkle over any remaining cilantro for decoration.

Corn fritters

MAKES AROUND 8 FRITTERS

2 large eggs
½ cup gluten-free flour
1 tsp baking powder
1 tbsp cornstarch
12oz canned corn, drained
2 scallions, coarsely chopped
1 tsp oat milk

1 tsp paprika
salt and pepper, to season
1 red chili, finely chopped
handful of cilantro, coarsely chopped
coconut oil, for cooking

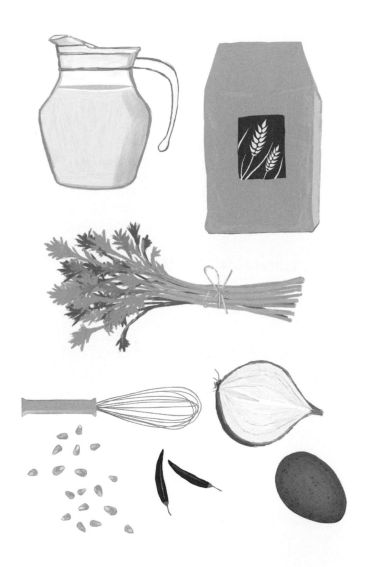

Serving suggestion

I like to serve with a poached egg, slices of avocado, and a drizzle of sweet chili sauce

Method

1. Beat the eggs in a large bowl. Add the flour, baking powder, cornstarch, corn, scallions, milk, and paprika, and mix through. Season with salt and pepper.

2. Transfer just over half the mixture to a food processor and blitz, before adding it back to the bowl of unblitzed mixture—again, stir through. Add the chili and cilantro to the mixture and season with salt and pepper.

3. Heat a little coconut oil in a skillet. Spoon even amounts of batter into the hot oil (this mix should make 8 fritters, but feel free to vary the size as you want). Cook for about 5 minutes on each side until crispy, then serve as suggested above.

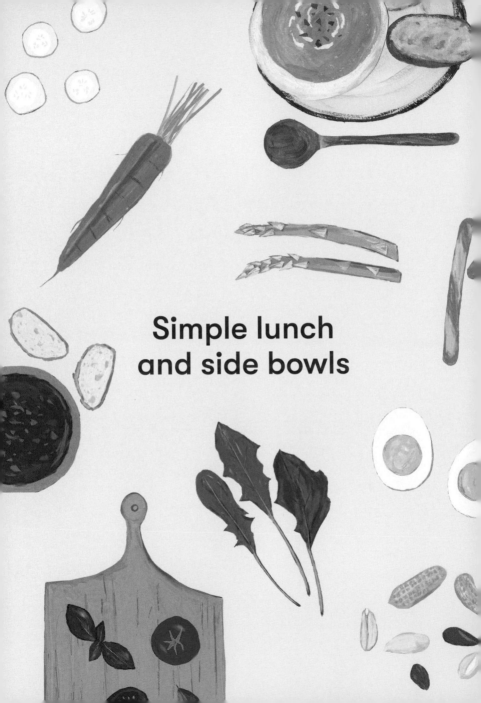

Simple lunch and side bowls

Carrot and coconut soup

SERVES 4

1 large sweet potato
1 white onion
1 tbsp coconut oil
1 red chili
3 garlic cloves
1 tsp fresh ginger, grated

4 carrots
14fl oz (1¾ cups) coconut milk
15fl oz vegetable stock
small handful cilantro, chopped
salt and pepper, to season

Method

1. Preheat the oven to 350°F (325°F convection).
2. Chop the sweet potato into small cubes. Place on a baking sheet, drizzle with oil, then pop in the oven and roast for 20 minutes.
3. Coarsely chop the onion, then place in a large pan and sauté in coconut oil until turning golden. Finely chop the chili and garlic, then add to the pan with the ginger. Coarsely chop the carrots, then add to the pan and cook for 3 more minutes. Add the coconut milk and stock. Bring to a boil for 5 minutes and then reduce to a simmer until the carrots are cooked.
4. When the sweet potato cubes are ready, add them to the pan along with the cilantro, and season with salt and pepper. Let cool slightly.
5. When the soup mix has cooled, transfer it to a blender and whizz it all together before returning to the pan to reheat. Bring to a boil to reduce and thicken to your preference.

Roasted red bell pepper and tomato soup

SERVES 4

4 red bell peppers

6 tomatoes, preferably on the vine

olive oil, for cooking

1 large white onion

2 carrots

2 medium baking potatoes

2 garlic cloves, finely diced

15fl oz vegetable stock

2 celery stalks

1 tbsp fresh basil, chopped

salt and pepper, to season

Method

1. Halve and seed the bell peppers and place on a baking sheet along with the tomatoes (include the stems if you're using tomatoes on the vine). Drizzle both with oil and roast for 15 minutes. Once cooked, set the bell peppers and tomatoes aside in a separate bowl to cool.

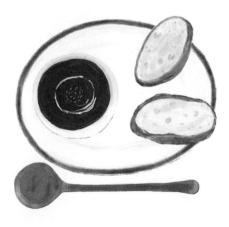

2. Coarsely chop the onion and sauté in olive oil in a large pan until golden. Coarsely chop the carrots and potatoes and add to the pan along with the garlic for an additional 5 minutes. Add the stock and bring to a boil. Coarsely chop and add the celery, then reduce the heat to a simmer.

3. Meanwhile, gently peel the skins off the red bell peppers and discard, so only the fleshy part is remaining. Mix all the ingredients together in a blender (include the tomato stems as they add a nice flavor to the soup—just make sure everything is fully blended).

4. Pour the soup back into the pan when fully blended to reheat. Add basil and season to taste.

Roasted pumpkin soup

SERVES 4

1 small pumpkin, seeded and coarsely chopped

1 sweet potato, coarsely diced

olive oil, for cooking

1 white onion, diced

2 garlic cloves, finely chopped

1 carrot, coarsely chopped

½ tsp ground cumin

½ tsp ground coriander

½ tsp ground cinnamon

3¾ cups vegetable stock

salt and pepper, to season

1 tbsp maple syrup

1 tbsp pumpkin seeds

Method

1. Preheat the oven to 350°F (325°F convection). Place the pumpkin and sweet potato onto a baking sheet, then drizzle with a little olive oil and a pinch of salt, and roast for 20–25 minutes until the flesh is soft.

2. Meanwhile, in a large pan, sauté the onion and garlic in a little

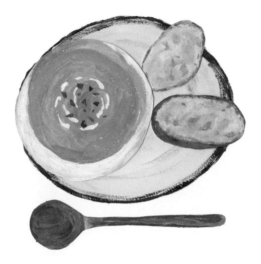

olive oil for a few minutes. Add the carrot and spices, then pour in the stock and bring to a boil, then lower the heat and simmer until the carrot is soft.

3. Add the roasted pumpkin and sweet potato to the pan and simmer for 2–3 more minutes. Transfer the mix to a blender and blitz until smooth and thick.

4. Taste, then season and add a drop of maple syrup, to suit your taste. To serve, drizzle maple syrup on top and scatter over a few pumpkin seeds.

Roasted tomato and basil soup

SERVES 4

12 large, plump, ripe tomatoes (select on the vine for better flavor)

olive oil, for cooking

1 white onion, diced

2 garlic cloves, finely diced

1 large carrot, coarsely chopped

14oz canned good-quality chopped tomatoes

2 cups vegetable stock

2 celery stalks, coarsely chopped

2 handfuls of basil

salt and pepper, to season

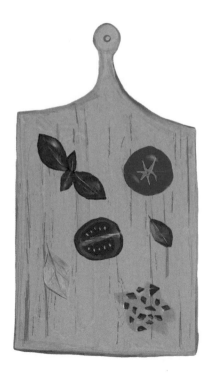

Method

1. Preheat the oven to 350°F (325°F convection). Place the fresh tomatoes on a baking sheet, then drizzle with oil and roast for about 20 minutes.

2. Meanwhile, sauté the onion in a pan with a little olive oil until turning golden, then add the garlic for 1 more minute. Add the carrot, canned tomatoes, and stock and bring to a boil for a few minutes, before turning the heat down. Add the celery, then simmer for another 5 minutes.

3. When the tomatoes are roasted, add them, along with the basil, to the pan and turn off the heat. Let cool down a little.

4. When cooled, transfer the soup to a blender and blitz for a couple of minutes. Season with salt and pepper and return to the stove to warm it up again to serve.

Pumpkin, kale, and pomegranate lunch bowl

SERVES 2

1 small pumpkin

4 tbsp olive oil

1 tbsp honey

7oz canned garbanzos, drained

1 tsp smoked paprika

salt and pepper, to season

2 generous handfuls of kale

1 tsp chili flakes

4 tbsp pine nuts or slivered almonds

seeds of ½ pomegranate

1 tbsp fresh parsley, chopped

Dressing

2 tbsp tahini

juice of 2 lemons

1 garlic clove, crushed and finely chopped

2 tbsp water

salt and pepper, to season

Method

1. Preheat the oven to 350°F (325°F convection). Slice the pumpkin into thick wedges (skin can remain on), removing all the seeds. Place on a baking sheet and drizzle with 2 tablespoons of olive oil and a tablespoon of honey. Roast for around 20–30 minutes, checking for when the flesh is tender.

2. Coat the garbanzos in 1 tablespoon of olive oil, paprika, and a pinch of salt and pepper. When the pumpkin has been in the oven for 10 minutes, take it out and scatter the garbanzos onto the same baking sheet. Then return the sheet to the oven to continue roasting.

3. In the meantime, make the dressing by mixing all the ingredients together in a bowl.

4. About 5 minutes before the pumpkin is ready, add the kale to the baking sheet and sprinkle with the remaining 1 tablespoon of olive oil, a pinch of salt and the chili flakes, then roast for 3–4 more minutes in the oven until crispy but not burned.

5. Toast the pine nuts or slivered almonds in a dry skillet on high heat for 2–3 minutes. Arrange the kale into two bowls, then scatter with the garbanzos and add the pumpkin wedges. Sprinkle pomegranate seeds, pine nuts or slivered almonds, and parsley over the bowl, then drizzle the dressing on top and serve warm.

Gado gado

SERVES 2

olive oil, for cooking

7oz tofu or tempeh, sliced

1 large white baking potato

2 eggs

1¼oz white cabbage, shredded

10 green beans, halved

2 tbsp bean sprouts

¼ cucumber, sliced into thin sticks

1 carrot, grated
1 tbsp peanuts, coarsely chopped
1 tbsp cilantro, coarsely chopped

juice of ½ lime
2 tbsp soy sauce
pinch of salt

Sauce
2 tbsp chunky peanut butter
1 red chili
1 garlic clove

Serving suggestion
serve with prawn chips

Method
1. Heat some oil and pan-fry the tofu or tempeh slices until they are light brown on both sides. Once cooked, place to one side on sheets of paper towel.

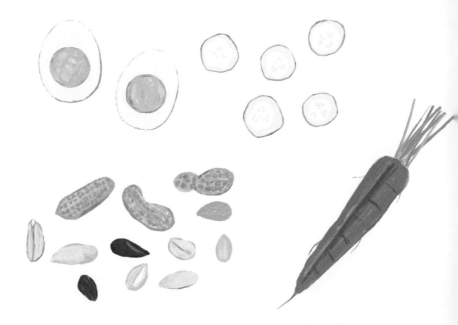

2. Chop the potato into neat little cubes and boil for just 3–4 minutes until soft (being careful not to over-boil). Hard-cook the eggs and cut them in half. Blanch the shredded cabbage in boiling water for 3 minutes. Blanch the green beans in boiling water until slightly tender but still crunchy.

3. Prepare the satay sauce by blending all the ingredients in a blender, or mix together with a spoon until it's fully combined—add a splash of water if you'd prefer a thinner consistency.

4. Drizzle the potato cubes with olive oil and season. Arrange the vegetables, tofu slices, and eggs into little piles in a bowl and drizzle with the satay sauce. Sprinkle with chopped peanuts and scatter over some cilantro.

Vegetable couscous salad

SERVES 2

6 decent-sized broccoli florets
6 decent-sized cauliflower florets
¼ red cabbage
2 celery stalks
2 corncobs
8oz halloumi (optional)
1 carrot, grated
1 scallion, finely chopped
2 tbsp seed mix
2 tbsp chopped almonds

1 ripe avocado, sliced
2 tbsp sprouting seeds
handful of cilantro, chopped
1 lime
pinch of salt

Serving suggestion
add a dollop of hummus
(see p.124)

Method

1. In a food processor, pulse the broccoli, cauliflower, cabbage, and celery together until it looks a bit like couscous.

2. Carefully place the corncobs in a pan of boiling water for 5 minutes, and pan-fry the halloumi (if using) on a low heat for a couple of minutes until golden brown on either side.

3. Add the grated carrot, chopped scallion, salad seeds, almonds, avocado, sprouting seeds, and cilantro to the vegetable "couscous." Squeeze a lime over it, then add a pinch of salt and mix together well.

4. Arrange the couscous mix into two bowls, sit the halloumi on top and the corncobs to the side. Sprinkle with any remaining cilantro.

Dips

Plain hummus

MAKES 1 SMALL DIPPING BOWL

14oz canned garbanzos, drained

3 garlic cloves

2 tbsp tahini

1 tsp ground cumin

½ tsp smoked paprika

1 tbsp vegan sour cream

juice of ½ lemon

pinch of salt

1 tsp olive oil

pinch of paprika

Method

Whizz all the ingredients together in a food processor. Transfer to a serving bowl and place in the refrigerator to chill. When you're ready to serve, drizzle olive oil over the hummus and add another pinch of paprika for decoration.

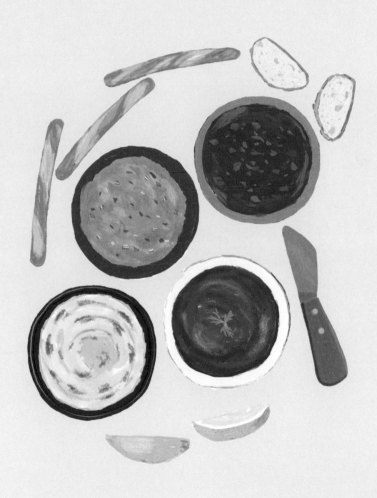

Beet hummus

MAKES 1 SMALL DIPPING BOWL

1 large beet, roasted

14oz canned garbanzos, drained

3 garlic cloves

2 tbsp tahini

1 tbsp vegan sour cream

juice of ½ lemon

pinch of salt

Method

Preheat the oven to 400°F (375°F convection). Roast the beet for about 1 hour. Once the beet is soft, whizz it with all the other ingredients in a food processor until smooth. Transfer to a serving bowl and place in the refrigerator to chill.

Guacamole

MAKES 1 SMALL DIPPING BOWL

3 ripe avocados

½ red onion

1 plump, ripe tomato

juice of ½ lime

1 tbsp cilantro, chopped

pinch of salt

Method

Scoop out the flesh of the avocados and add to a mixing bowl. Dice the red onion very finely and add to the bowl. Finely chop the tomato and add to the bowl. Squeeze the lime juice into the bowl and add the cilantro, plus a pinch of salt. Mix it all together with a fork.

Salsa

MAKES 1 SMALL DIPPING BOWL

6 plump tomatoes, on the vine
piece of cucumber (about 3¼in)
½ red onion
1 large red chili (add more or less
to suit taste)

1 tbsp cilantro, chopped
pinch of salt

Method

Chop the tomato and cucumber into small, neat, equal-size cubes. Finely chop the red onion and chili. Combine everything together in a mixing bowl, adding the cilantro and a pinch of salt.

Asparagus, spinach, and pea risotto

SERVES 4 AS A SIDE OR APPETIZER, OR 2 AS A MAIN COURSE

good chunk of butter (or dairy-
free spread)
6 asparagus stems, halved
1 large onion, chopped
2 garlic cloves, chopped
11½oz (1½ cups) risotto rice
½ cup dry white wine (optional)
3 pints vegetable stock

½ cup frozen peas
½ cup grated Parmesan cheese (or
Parma vegan)
3 full handfuls of spinach greens
salt and pepper, to season
1 sprig fresh rosemary, finely chopped

Method

1. Add a small amount of the butter to a skillet and sauté the asparagus stems on high heat until slightly brown but not overcooked, then put to one side.

2. In a separate skillet, heat the rest of the butter until melted. Add the onion and garlic and stir for 2 minutes. Stir in the rice for 2 minutes until completely coated in butter. If you are using wine, add this now and keep stirring until it has been totally absorbed by the rice.

3. Start to slowly add the stock, one ladle at a time, letting it be absorbed by the rice and then adding more, stirring continuously. This should take around 20 minutes. Before the last ladle goes in, add the peas and stir through half the Parmesan cheese. Add the last ladle of stock and the spinach and keep stirring. Once all the liquid has been absorbed, add salt and pepper to taste, along with the rosemary and the remaining Parmesan cheese.

4. Place the asparagus pan back onto really high heat to warm through. Spoon the risotto mix into bowls, then arrange the asparagus on top and scatter over any remaining rosemary.

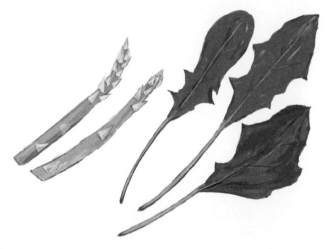

Red lentil and cauliflower dal

SERVES 4 AS A SIDE OR APPETIZER, OR 2 AS A MAIN COURSE

1 tbsp coconut oil
1 large white onion, finely chopped
3 garlic cloves, crushed and finely chopped
1 tsp ground cumin
1 tsp ground coriander
1 tsp ground turmeric
1 tsp garam masala
3½oz cauliflower florets, chopped into small pieces

14fl oz (1¾ cups) coconut milk
2 cups vegetable stock
7oz (1 cup) red lentils
2 generous handfuls of spinach
handful of cilantro, chopped
salt, for seasoning

Serving suggestion
serve with rice or naan bread

Method

1. Heat the coconut oil in a skillet and sauté the onion until golden. Add the garlic and spices and mix well for 1 minute. Add the cauliflower and stir until coated in the spice mix. Add the coconut milk and stock, along with the lentils, and bring to a boil.

2. Lower the heat to a simmer, stirring occasionally, for around 20 minutes, until the lentils are cooked and the mixture is thick. Add the spinach and cilantro and mix well until the spinach has wilted. Season to taste and serve hot.

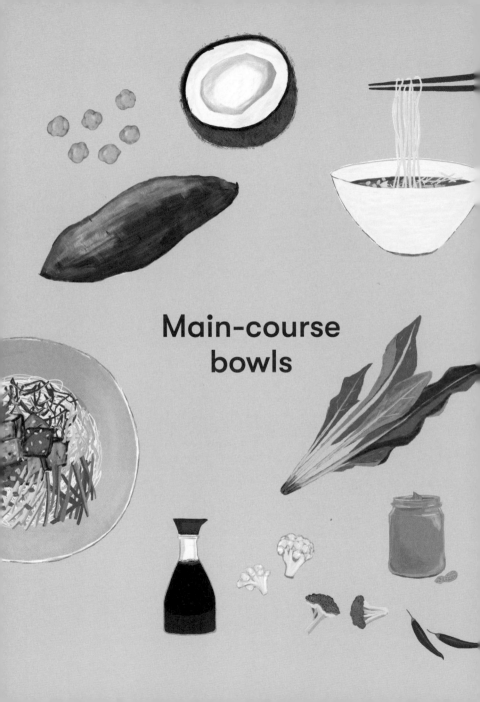

Main-course bowls

Ramen

SERVES 2

10oz tofu

coconut oil, for cooking

1 medium white onion, sliced

1 red chili (adjust amount
according to taste)

3 garlic cloves, finely chopped

2 tsp fresh ginger, chopped

1 tbsp miso paste

1 tbsp sesame oil

18fl oz (1¼ pints) vegetable stock

3 tbsp soy sauce

10 mushrooms, sliced

1 medium carrot, sliced

6 pieces baby corn, sliced in
half lengthwise

2 nests rice noodles

1 head bok choy, separated into leaves
and trimmed

handful of cilantro, coarsely chopped

1oz (or 2 handfuls) bean sprouts

1 scallion, chopped into 2in pieces

1 tbsp sesame seeds

Method

1. Preheat the oven to 400°F (375°F convection). Slice the tofu lengthwise into strips, then drizzle with coconut oil (if solid, warm in a pan before drizzling) and place on a baking sheet in the oven for 20 minutes, turning them over halfway.

2. In a wok, stir-fry the onion, chili, and garlic in coconut oil for 2–3 minutes. Add the ginger, miso, sesame oil, stock, and soy sauce, bring to a boil and simmer for around 5 minutes.

3. To suit your preference, either strain the broth into another pan and discard the remaining onion and ginger, or just leave them in. Add the mushrooms and carrot, then bring back to a boil and simmer for 3 minutes.

4. When the tofu has 10 minutes of cooking time left, and needs turning over, add the baby corn to the baking sheet and drizzle with sesame oil. Roast together for the remaining 10 minutes.

4. Cook the rice noodles according to the package directions and divide between two bowls when ready.

5. Add the bok choy and cilantro to the broth. Taste and adjust as necessary to suit your preference (does it need more chili, garlic, or herbs?). Once the bok choy has started to wilt, pour the broth evenly into the two bowls, over the noodles.

6. Arrange a handful of bean sprouts, cooked tofu, and baby corn around the edge of the bowl. Then sprinkle the chopped scallions, cilantro and sesame seeds over the dish, and serve.

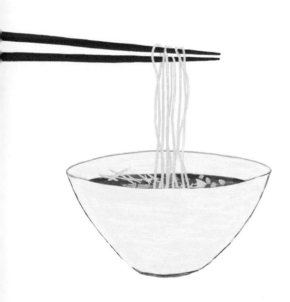

Poke bowl

SERVES 2

5oz white or brown rice

sesame oil, for cooking

10oz tofu, cubed

1 ripe avocado, sliced

1 carrot, grated

2 tbsp fresh edamame beans

4 radishes, sliced

2 tbsp instant wakame or shredded
Napa cabbage

Flesh from 1 fresh mango, cubed

2 tsp pickled ginger

1 tbsp sesame seeds

Satay sauce

2 tbsp dark soy sauce

1 tbsp hot water

2 tbsp peanut butter

2 tbsp sweet chili sauce

1 garlic clove, finely chopped

juice of ½ lime

Method

1. Cook the rice according to the package directions, then set aside to cool.

2. Mix all the sauce ingredients together in a bowl. Taste and adjust to suit your preference, and then set to one side.

3. Heat the oil in a skillet and cook the cubed chunks of tofu for 10 minutes, turning and stirring to ensure all sides turn brown and crispy.

4. Divide the cooked rice between two bowls. Arrange the sliced avocado, grated carrot, edamame beans, sliced radish, wakame, mango, and pickled ginger decoratively around each bowl, then add the cooked tofu.

5. Sprinkle sesame seeds and drizzle the satay dressing over both bowls.

Sweet and zingy buddha bowl

SERVES 2

1 sweet potato, cut into wedges

olive oil, for cooking and drizzling

1 tsp honey

1 corncob

2 carrots, grated

2 tbsp sesame seeds

handful of cilantro, chopped

juice of ½ lime

juice of ½ lemon

6oz (scant 1 cup) cooked lentils

2 cooked beet, cut into little cubes

2 tbsp red cabbage, shredded

5 radishes, sliced

1 avocado, sliced

handful of salad greens

10 cherry tomatoes, halved

dollop of hummus (see page 124)

Dressing

2 tbsp olive oil

juice of ½ lemon

salt and pepper, to season

Serving suggestion

Add broiled halloumi or tofu

Method

1. Preheat the oven to 350°F (325°F convection). Place the sweet potato wedges on a baking sheet, coat with olive oil and honey, then roast in the oven for 25–30 minutes.

2. Submerge the corn in boiling water for 5 minutes, and when cooked, set aside to cool.

3. Place the grated carrot into a bowl and sprinkle over 1 tablespoon of the sesame seeds, most of the chopped cilantro and the juice from half a lime. Mix in the lentils and beet, a drizzle of olive oil, and juice from half a lemon, and season.

4. Mix together the ingredients for your dressing.

5. In a flattish bowl, start to arrange your buddha bowl ingredients. Spoon your carrot, lentil, and beet mix, shredded cabbage, radish, avocado, salad greens, and cherry tomatoes into little piles. Slice the corn from the cob lengthwise and add to your bowl.

6. When the sweet-potato wedges are cooked, transfer them hot to your bowl. Add a dollop of hummus in the center of the bowl and spoon the dressing over the whole bowl to taste. Sprinkle the remaining cilantro and sesame seeds, and serve.

Nasi goreng

SERVES 2

1 cup brown rice

2 tbsp coconut oil

1 large white onion, diced

4 garlic cloves, finely chopped

1 fresh chili, finely chopped

1 carrot, diced

4 medium broccoli florets, cut into fourths

4 medium cauliflower florets, cut into fourths

2 large handfuls of fresh kale or spinach

4½oz (1⅓ cups) frozen peas

salt and pepper, to season

2 tbsp peanut butter

4 tbsp soy sauce

1 tbsp tomato paste

1 tbsp sweet chili sauce (or replace with maple syrup and 1 extra fresh chili)

2 tbsp cashews

1 tbsp mixed seeds

2 eggs

bunch of cilantro, coarsely chopped

Serving suggestion

1 scallion, sliced

drizzle of sriracha

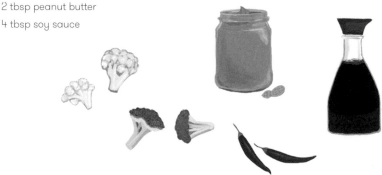

Method

1. Boil the rice according to the package directions.

2. Heat the coconut oil in a skillet and sauté the onion for 5 minutes until golden. Add the chopped garlic and chili and cook for 1 more minute. Add the carrot, broccoli, and cauliflower and cook for 3–4 minutes. Add the kale and peas, then season and cook for another 3–4 minutes.

3. Meanwhile, mix together the peanut butter, soy sauce, tomato paste, and sweet chili sauce in a bowl, with a splash of boiling water.

4. When the rice is cooked, add it to the vegetable mix along with the cashews and mixed seeds and combine. Pour the sauce mixture over the rice and vegetables in the skillet, thoroughly stir it all through and cook for an additional 2–3 minutes.

5. In a separate skillet, fry the two eggs. Just before serving, add the cilantro to the nasi goreng mix in the skillet and stir through.

6. To serve, divide the rice mixture between two bowls, and top each one with a fried egg. Then sprinkle over the scallion with any leftover bits of chili, and a drizzle of sriracha.

Apricot tagine

SERVES 2

3 parsnips (or 1 large baking potato if you'd prefer), cubed

olive oil, for cooking

salt and pepper, to season

1 large white onion, diced

2 large garlic cloves, diced

1 heaping tsp harissa paste

1 tsp fresh ginger, grated or chopped

1 tsp ground coriander

½ tsp ground turmeric

1 tsp ground cinnamon

½ red bell pepper, sliced

1 carrot, diced

1 tsp tomato paste

scant 1¼ cups vegetable stock

1lb 12oz canned good-quality
chopped tomatoes

10 dried apricots

7oz canned garbanzos, drained

bunch of cilantro, chopped

½ lemon (optional)

Serving suggestion

serve with couscous, quinoa, rice, or
bread

Method

1. Preheat the oven to 350°F (325°F convection).
2. Put the parsnips (or potatoes) on a baking sheet, drizzle with oil, then season and place in the oven for 12–15 minutes.
3. Meanwhile, sauté the onion in a drizzle of olive oil until turning golden. Add the garlic, harissa paste, ginger, and spices and mix through.
4. Add the red bell pepper, carrot, and tomato paste, then season with salt and pepper, and stir for a couple of minutes. Add the stock and chopped tomatoes and mix together well.
5. Add the dried apricots, roasted parsnips, garbanzos and 2 teaspoons of fresh, chopped cilantro, and stir everything together. Turn down the heat, then cover and simmer for 20 minutes until the consistency is thick and the vegetables are cooked.
6. Taste before serving and adjust the flavors to suit your preference—for example, by adding a squeeze of lemon juice, a bit more harissa, or some more seasoning.
7. Dish up into bowls, sprinkled with some more freshly chopped cilantro. Serve with couscous, quinoa, rice, or bread.

Sweet potato and coconut curry

SERVES 2

1 sweet potato

olive oil, for cooking

2 tbsp coconut oil

1 large white onion, finely chopped

3 garlic cloves, finely chopped

1 red chili, finely chopped

1 tsp ground coriander

1 tsp garam masala

1 tsp ground turmeric

1 tbsp curry powder

14fl oz (1¾ cups) coconut milk

7oz canned good-quality chopped tomatoes

2 handfuls of spinach

7oz canned garbanzos, drained

1 tbsp peanut butter

1 tbsp dry unsweetened coconut

handful of cilantro, chopped

7oz (1 cup) brown rice

pinch of salt

Method

1. Preheat the oven to 350°F (325°F convection). Cut the sweet potato into small cubes, then drizzle with olive oil and roast in the oven for around 20 minutes.

2. Heat the coconut oil in a large wok or skillet and sauté the onion until golden. Add the garlic and chili and cook for another 1 minute. Add the ground coriander, garam masala, turmeric, and curry powder and cook for 1 more minute.

3. Add the coconut milk and mix well with the curry paste you've made in the pan. Add the canned tomatoes, mixing well, and bring the whole pan to a boil for a few minutes, then reduce to a simmer.

4. Once the sweet potatoes are roasted through, add them to the curry mix along with a handful of spinach, the garbanzos and peanut butter, and half a tablespoon of the desiccated coconut. Add a handful of cilantro (keeping a small amount to one side to garnish), then cover the whole mix and simmer for as long as possible until it is nice and thick.

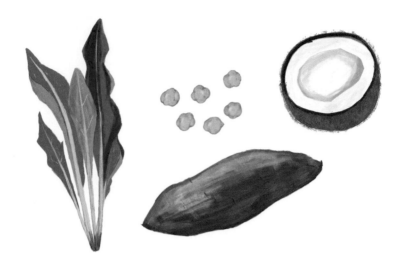

5. A half-hour before you want to serve, cook the brown rice according to package directions. When the rice is cooked, mix the remaining half tablespoon of dry unsweetened coconut and the second handful of spinach through the rice, with a pinch of salt.

6. Taste and adjust to suit your preference (does it need more chili, coconut, garlic, or peanut butter?). Serve over the rice. Add the remaining fresh chopped cilantro to the curry to garnish.

Katsu curry

SERVES 2

Crispy tofu

1 tbsp cornstarch

2 tbsp water

10oz tofu, sliced into strips

2 tbsp crispy bread crumbs

olive oil, for cooking

Curry sauce

coconut oil, for cooking

1 large white onion, finely chopped

3 garlic cloves, chopped

1 tsp fresh ginger, grated

1 tbsp mild curry powder

½ red chili, chopped

1 tsp ground turmeric

1 tsp ground coriander

1 tsp garam masala

4 medium to large carrots, coarsely chopped

1 tbsp maple syrup

14fl oz (1¾ cups) coconut milk

scant 1¼ cups vegetable stock

handful of cilantro, chopped

pinch of salt

Serving suggestion

serve with jasmine rice

Method

1. Preheat the oven to 375°F (350°F convection).

2. Mix the cornstarch and water together in a bowl. Dip the tofu strips into the cornstarch mix to lightly coat before dipping into bread crumbs, fully covering each tofu strip. Place on a baking sheet, then drizzle with olive oil and roast for 20 minutes, turning a few times.

3. Heat the coconut oil in a large pan. Add the onion for a couple of minutes until turning golden. Add the garlic, ginger, curry powder, chili, turmeric, ground coriander, and garam masala, and stir through to make a curry paste. Add the carrots, maple syrup, coconut milk, and stock, and bring to a boil. Lower to a simmer until the carrots are starting to soften.

4. Add a tablespoon of chopped cilantro and a pinch of salt, and transfer the whole mix to a blender to blitz for 4–5 minutes until the curry sauce is silky smooth.

5. Transfer the sauce back to the pan and taste—make any adjustments to suit your own personal taste by adding a little more spice, coriander, garlic, or seasoning.

6. Take the crispy tofu out of the oven. Divide equally between two bowls, then add the rice and pour the curry sauce over the top, garnishing with the remaining cilantro.

Pad Thai

SERVES 2

2 nests flat rice noodles

coconut oil, for cooking

1 large white onion, sliced

4 garlic cloves, chopped

1 red chili, finely chopped (add more chili to taste)

7oz bean sprouts

5 long-stem broccoli stems, chopped into smaller pieces

1 carrot, chopped into thin small strips

pinch of salt

2 tbsp dark soy sauce

2 tbsp fish sauce (replace with soy sauce to make vegan)

1 tbsp rice wine

1 tbsp sweet chili sauce

1 tbsp maple syrup

2 limes

1 tbsp peanut butter

3 eggs, beaten

2 tbsp coarsely chopped peanuts

handful of cilantro, chopped

1 scallion, chopped

Method

1. Partially cook the noodles and set aside (boil them just a few minutes shy of the cooking directions found on the package—this is to ensure the noodles don't shred into pieces when they are added to the dish later on in the recipe).

2. Heat the coconut oil in a large skillet or wok. Sauté the onion, garlic, and chilli for a couple of minutes. Add the bean sprouts, broccoli, and carrot, then add a pinch of salt and cook for another 2–3 minutes.

3. Add the soy sauce, fish sauce, rice wine, sweet chili sauce, and maple syrup, then squeeze in the juice of one of the limes and mix through. Add the peanut butter, scattering it in little chunks around the skillet.

4. Add the part-cooked noodles and mix the whole lot through, adding a dash more coconut oil if needed, for 2–3 minutes.

5. Push the noodle mix over to one side of the skillet and pour the beaten egg into the other side, stirring occasionally to form large chunks of scrambled egg.

6. Once the scrambled egg has formed, add a tablespoon of chopped peanuts and most of the cilantro, then stir the whole mix together. Taste and adjust to suit your preference.

7. Serve into two bowls and sprinkle remaining cilantro, chopped scallion, the rest of the chopped peanuts, and any remaining chili over the top of the dish. Garnish with a wedge of lime.

Vietnamese noodle bowl

SERVES 2

7oz smoked tofu

1 tbsp sesame oil

2 nests vermicelli noodles

1¼oz red cabbage, shredded

4 lettuce leaves, shredded

1 carrot, cut into thin strips

piece of cucumber (about 4in), cut into thin strips

1 scallion, green end, sliced

1 tbsp white and black sesame seeds

handful of cilantro, finely chopped

Dressing

5 tbsp rice vinegar

juice of 1 lime

3 tbsp dark soy sauce

2 tbsp maple syrup

1 red chili, chopped (adjust amount according to taste)

1 garlic clove, finely chopped

1 scallion, white end, chopped

1 tbsp cilantro, chopped

Method

1. Preheat the oven to 400°F (375°F convection).

2. Mix all the dressing ingredients together in a small bowl and set aside.

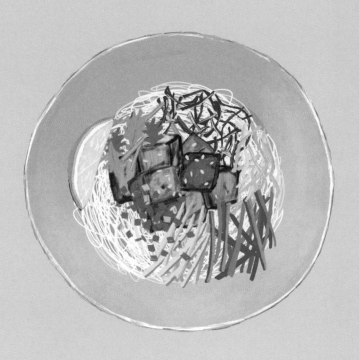

3. Cut the tofu into little cubes, then coat them in sesame oil and place on a baking sheet in the oven for 20 minutes, turning and moving them around the sheet occasionally.

4. Cook the noodles according to the package directions. Once cooked, divide the noodles between two bowls. Arrange the shredded cabbage, lettuce, carrot, and cucumber around the bowls, and add the baked tofu.

5. Drizzle over the dressing, and sprinkle the sliced green end of the scallion over the bowls, along with the sesame seeds. Garnish with cilantro and serve.

Mexican frijoles

SERVES 4

1 white onion

4 garlic cloves

olive oil, for cooking

2 red chiles

1 tsp ground cumin

1 cup vegetable stock

1lb 12oz canned black beans or pinto beans, drained

1 bay leaf

Salsa

6 tomatoes

1 red onion

1 cucumber

1 large handful of cilantro

salt and pepper, to season

To serve

7oz bag of corn nachos

5fl oz ($^1/_3$ cup) tub vegan sour cream

Method

1. Finely chop the onion and garlic, then place in a skillet, and sauté in olive oil until turning brown. Chop one of the chiles and add to the pan, along with the cumin, and mix together for 1–2 minutes. Add the stock, beans, and bay leaf, and bring to a boil for 5 minutes. Then, reduce the heat to a simmer and cook for an additional 25 minutes, stirring occasionally.

2. Meanwhile, make the salsa. Finely dice the tomatoes into small cubes and transfer to a bowl. Finely dice the red onion and cucumber and add. Finely chop 1 handful of cilantro, then add to the salsa and season.

3. When the stock has boiled down and the beans are soft, taste and adjust to suit your preference (adding more spice, garlic, or seasoning) before spooning the frijoles mix into bowls. Add a spoonful of the salsa and sour cream. Serve with the nachos and a dipping bowl of any leftover salsa.

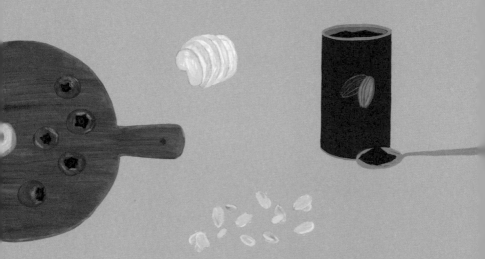

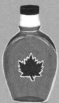

Dessert Bowls

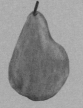

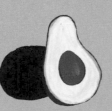

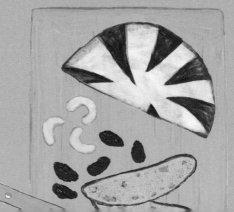

Raw caramel slices

SERVES 4–6

Base
²/₃ cup almonds
2 tbsp dry unsweetened coconut
8 pitted dates
4 tbsp melted coconut oil

Caramel
10 pitted Medjool dates
4 tbsp cashew-nut butter

1 tsp vanilla extract
4 tbsp maple syrup
pinch of salt

Topping
3 tbsp melted coconut oil
2 tbsp maple syrup
6 tbsp raw cacao powder

Method
1. Mix all the ingredients for the base together in a food processor until blended and crumbly. Press the mixture into the base of a 6in cake pan and place in the freezer while you make the caramel.
2. To make the "caramel," mix all the ingredients in a food processor until really smooth and soft. Spread the caramel over the prepared base and return to the freezer while you make the topping.
3. For the topping, melt the oil in a heatproof bowl over a pan of simmering water. Add the maple syrup, then add the cacao powder and mix together until smooth.
4. Pour the topping mixture over the caramel and place in the refrigerator for at least 2 hours until set. Slice into bite-size pieces for a snack, or larger dessert-size slices.

Vegan chocolate mousse

SERVES 2 AS A MINI PUDDING

1 super-ripe avocado (but make
sure the flesh is beautifully green,
not brown)
3 tbsp maple syrup

1 tbsp honey
4 tbsp cacao powder
2 tbsp oat milk or coconut milk
1 tbsp vegan sour cream

Method

1. Blend the flesh of the avocado, maple syrup, honey, cacao
powder, milk, and sour cream in a small food processor, until thick
and super-smooth.
2. Separate the mixture into two small glasses or ramekins. Place in
the refrigerator for a couple of hours (or longer) before serving.

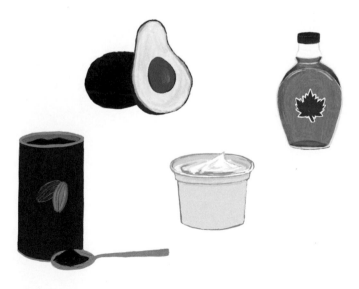

Indonesian black rice pudding

SERVES 4

½ cup black rice

7fl oz water

14fl oz (1¾ cups) coconut milk

2 tbsp maple syrup

2 tbsp dry unsweetened coconut

pinch of salt

2 tbsp coconut yogurt

Method

1. Add the black rice to a pan with the water, coconut milk, 1 tablespoon of the maple syrup, and 1 tablespoon of dry unsweetened coconut, and bring to the boil.

2. Lower the heat to a simmer, then cover and cook for 35–40 minutes, occasionally stirring and adding a splash more water if needed. It should reduce down to a thick consistency.

3. When the rice is tender and the consistency thick, add the other tablespoon of maple syrup, a tablespoon of dry unsweetened coconut, and a pinch of salt, and mix through.

4. Separate into bowls and top with a dollop of coconut yogurt and a sprinkling of the remaining dry unsweetened coconut.

Raw vegan blueberry cheesecake

SERVES 4–6

Base

12 pitted dates

6oz (1¾ cups) walnuts

Filling

1 cup raw cashews

3 tbsp honey

2 tbsp coconut oil

6 tbsp coconut yogurt

3½oz (²/₃ cup) blueberries

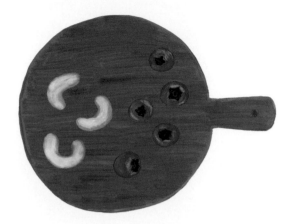

Method

1. Pulse the dates and walnuts together in a blender and transfer the mixture to 4–6 small ramekins or glasses; pack it right down to form the base.

2. Whizz the cashews, honey, coconut oil, yogurt, and blueberries in the blender, then spoon the mixture evenly over the base.

3. Cover with foil or plastic wrap and place in the refrigerator for around 5 hours before serving.

Vegan crème brûlée

SERVES 2–3

14fl oz (1¾ cups) coconut milk

1 tbsp corn starch

2 tbsp maple syrup

1 tsp vanilla extract

pinch of sea salt

2 tsp coconut sugar (or cane sugar)

Serving suggestion

serve with berries of your choice

Method

1. Blitz all the ingredients together in a blender until really smooth.
2. Transfer the mixture to a small pan and start to simmer, stirring until it becomes a thicker, creamy consistency.
3. Transfer to separate ramekins and let cool, then place in the refrigerator for a couple of hours to set.
4. When you are ready to serve, sprinkle the top with sugar and place under the broiler for a couple of minutes (or use a kitchen torch), until it starts to caramelize and crisp up. As a serving suggestion, top with a few berries of your choice.

Coconut poached pears

SERVES 2

14fl oz (1¾ cups) coconut milk
2 tbsp maple syrup
1 tsp vanilla extract
1 tsp ground cinnamon
1 tbsp coconut sugar

1 tbsp water
4 pears, skinned (but leave the stem on)
2 tbsp coconut yogurt
1 tbsp slivered almonds

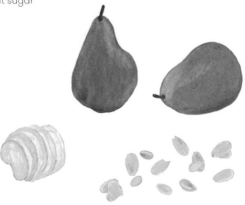

Method

1. Add the coconut milk, maple syrup, vanilla extract, cinnamon, sugar, and water to a pan and bring to a boil. Add the pears, then cover and reduce to a simmer.

2. After about 30 minutes, check on the pears: they should be soft, but keep simmering for 5 more minutes.

3. When cooked, divide the pears between two bowls. Top with coconut yogurt, slivered almonds, and a sprinkling of cinnamon.

Vegan bread pudding

SERVES 4

scant 2½ cups creamy oat milk

4 tbsp coconut yogurt

2 tsp ground cinnamon

4 tbsp cashews

1 tsp vanilla extract

4 tbsp maple syrup

2 tbsp coconut sugar

2 tbsp raisins

1 small loaf sourdough (or gluten-free) bread

coconut cream, to serve

Method

1. Preheat the oven to 350°F (325°F convection).

2. Blend the oat milk, 4 tablespoons of yogurt, cinnamon, cashews, vanilla extract, maple syrup, and 1 tablespoon of the coconut sugar in a blender until smooth. Add the whole raisins to the batter mix.

3. Slice the loaf of bread into thick slices, and layer them into an ovenproof dish or separate ramekins, pouring a little of the liquid mixture over each layer of bread.

4. Sprinkle the remaining tablespoon of coconut sugar over the top layer of bread. Transfer to the oven and bake for 45 minutes. Serve with a dollop of coconut cream on top.

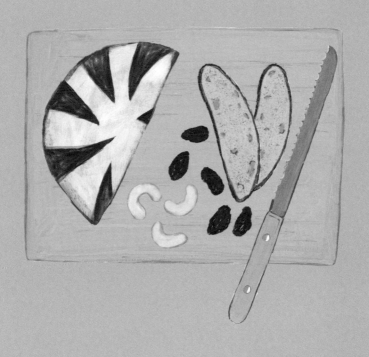

Lucy's vegan, sugar-free carrot cake

MAKES 12 SLICES

3 tbsp flax seed

6 tbsp orange juice

¾ cup vegan spread

²/₃ cup coconut sugar

zest and juice of 1 orange

¾ cup self-rising flour

1 tsp baking powder

pinch of sea salt

1 tsp allspice

generous ¾ cup ground almonds

generous ¹/₃ cup golden raisins

2¾oz mixed seeds

9oz carrots, finely grated

Topping

8fl oz (1 cup) coconut cream

1 tsp vanilla extract

2 tbsp coconut sugar

1 tbsp mixed seeds to finish

Method

1. Preheat the oven to 350°F (325°F convection). Line 2 × 8in sandwich pans with parchment paper.

2. Prepare the topping by whisking together all ingredients, except the seeds, until light and fluffy, then pop in the refrigerator for a couple of minutes until it's a spreadable consistency.

3. Mix the flax seed with the 6 tablespoons of orange juice in a small mixing bowl, and set aside to sit for a couple of minutes.

4. Beat together the vegan spread, coconut sugar, and orange juice and zest to a cream. Add the flax-seed mixture, flour, baking powder, salt, and allspice to the bowl, and mix well. Fold in the ground almonds, golden raisins, seeds, and grated carrot.

5. Divide the mixture between the two prepared pans and bake for 40 minutes until even in color and springy to touch. Take the cakes out of the oven and let them stand in the pans for 10 minutes before turning out onto a cooling rack.

6. When the cake is cold, sandwich half the topping between the

two layers and spread the other half on top. Finish with mixed seeds. Keep in an airtight container for up to 4 days.

Peanut bites

MAKES 12 BITES

2 tbsp coconut oil

4 tbsp cacao powder

2 tbsp maple syrup

12 pitted dates

1 tbsp peanut butter

1 tbsp dry unsweetened coconut

Method

1. Melt the coconut oil, then make the chocolate sauce by mixing the oil with the cacao powder and maple syrup.

2. Carefully stuff each date with a little bit of peanut butter. Roll them in the chocolate sauce, before placing onto a sheet of parchment paper or a plate.

3. Sprinkle a little dry unsweetened coconut over the top and pop in the refrigerator for a couple of hours.

Coconut and lime bites

MAKES 12 BITES

1 cup cashews

1 tsp maple syrup

3½oz (generous ½ cup) pitted dates

3 tbsp dry unsweetened coconut

3 drops almond extract

juice of ½ lime

Pulse all the ingredients in a food processor. Roll into small, bite-size balls. Keep in the refrigerator until you are ready to serve.

Closing thoughts

A mindful eating practice does not mean being perfect, righteous, or making the "right" choice every time. It isn't about denying yourself what you enjoy, subscribing to a diet, or judging yourself or others for food choices. Instead, it involves being curious and compassionate in your relationship with food. It is about love.

For those of us who have the privilege of choice, the food we eat is who we are and it is a relationship between us and the earth. A mindful eating practice reminds us to be present; and, from that state of presence, it is often easier to choose food that will balance our gut microbiome, give us energy, and contribute to a thriving, well-functioning mind and body, rather than foods that will deplete us of energy, give us brain fog, and give our body more work to do.

A mindful eating practice can help us identify, with the deepest compassion, if we need help and support in building a healthier relationship with food, and with ourselves.

Food is a pleasureful, earthly gift and cooking is alchemy. Recipes tell a story of culture, family, and of self, while our eating habits teach us about our values and our relationship with ourselves. A mindful eating practice helps us to pay attention, listen, tend to, and learn. Thus, paired with the right intention, food becomes a tool for self-care, connection, and love.

You deserve to eat well and really enjoy the foods you love. The planet deserves, in this era of choice, plenty, and opportunity, that we do so mindfully and take responsibility for choosing consciously and compassionately where we can.

As conscious consumers, we must also remember that the choices we make affect others, too. They not only have an impact on our family, our local community, and our economy but also on families and communities on the other side of the world as well. Our choices, however small, have an effect on the environment and this beautiful planet we call home. The food we eat is political, and it affects our individual and collective health; we quite simply have a responsibility to be considerate, even when it would be much more convenient for us to turn a blind eye.

Mindful eating is just one area of focus in a much broader mindfulness practice. By practicing with one activity—in this case, with food and eating—it can create a domino effect, enabling us to embody a state of presence and live more consciously, in other areas of our lives too. Creating rituals around our intentions and activities can help create a structure within which these intentions are more likely to be upheld. All you need to do is simply start right where you are, be flexible and kind to yourself—and grateful that most of us do have the privilege of choice.

I hope you have found this book to be a grateful celebration of food, glorious food! And I hope you feel supported and encouraged to be curious and compassionate, to go a little slower, to really taste, savor, and enjoy the food you eat. I hope you have some fun bringing these simple, home-cooking recipes to life. Be sure to share your creations with me on Instagram, tagging @joeyhulin_writer #mindandbowl if you do.

For now, I invite you to remember that old saying "Cooking is love made visible" and to choose love.

Index

Author acknowledgments

This book was first written and self-published as a pocketbook back in 2016, after New Year's Eve Retreat guests made me promise I would write down a few recipes, alongside some of the mindful eating guidance we had discussed on the retreat. A couple of weeks later, on my birthday in early January, I went for dinner with a dear friend, Frances Verbeek, who presented me with a voucher. She gifted me a couple of hours of her design time, to help me (a non-designer) bring the book to life. Knowing how much I need, and thrive on, a deadline, the voucher also featured the rather pressing and urgent deadline of the end of February. That evening I wrote the name of the book on a napkin and posted a photo on Instagram, for extra accountability, before clearing my schedule, shutting myself away, and having the time of my life writing *The Little Book of Mindful Eating*. My aunty, Claire David, kindly gifted her time to act as editor for that first edition. That early experience confirmed with every fiber of my being that writing books lights me up, brings me purpose, and is a process I utterly adore, from start to finish. Never in a million years did I think that that little book would one day transform, grow wings, and become this—*Mind and Bowl*.

I am forever grateful to commissioning editor Zara Larcombe for giving me the opportunity to write *Mind and Bowl* and to editor Chelsea Edwards for being so fantastic to work with! It takes such an immense amount of teamwork to bring a book to life, and I am grateful to all at Laurence King who were involved in this book. I had the incredible good fortune of writing this book in some utterly unique and breath-taking spaces, thanks to the kindness and generosity of others. Thank you to the ever-generous Karen Wells West, at The Sanctuary Cornwall in Golant, for letting me set up a little writing desk for a week-long writing retreat, tapping away at my laptop with the backdrop of sweeping river views. Thank you to Clare Fortescue for welcoming me to Boconnoc House in Cornwall, where I spent three glorious weeks tucked away in the library, surrounded by books and the romance and poetry of the place. A heartfelt thank you to Julie Tamblyn for letting me base myself at one of my favorite places on the planet, Botelet Cornwall, where I wrote the majority of this book. Thank you to Tia and Richard Tamblyn, for kindly offering their inspiring, grounded, and amusing reflections on the importance of family eating in chapter 5, and for being who they are.

Thank you to friends (and now professional recipe testers!) Jess North, Liz Kingdon, Rebecca Spurrier, Julie Moss, Lucinda Walton, Lisa Allen, Poppy Richards, Susie Petherick, Lisa Grigsby, and Mel Connell for playing with the recipes found in this book and for their invaluable feedback. Thank you to Lucy O'Hagan for contributing her insanely delicious cake recipe found on page 154 and for being such an incredible friend to me over the years. Thank you to my mum, Nikki Hulin, for her time, consistent support, and championing of all my work, and to all my dear friends who do the same. Thank you to my soul sister and the best writer I know, Frida Stavenow, for reading and feeding back her thoughts on this book.

Finally, a huge thank you to those 2016/17 New Year retreat guests for that original nudge, and all those who have attended, worked on, and been a part of the Horizon Inspired over the years—it is a joy.